Run. Walk. Eat.

CARISSA GALLOWAY RDN • JEFF GALLOWAY

RUN. WALK. EAT.

A Practical Nutrition Guide to Help Runners and Walkers
Improve Their Performance and Maximize Their Health

Meyer & Meyer Sport

British Library of Cataloguing in Publication Data
A catalogue record for this book is available from the British Library

Run. Walk. Eat.
Maidenhead: Meyer & Meyer Sport (UK) Ltd., 2024
ISBN: 978-1-78255-261-1

© 2024 by Meyer & Meyer Sport (UK) Ltd.
Aachen, Auckland, Beirut, Cairo, Cape Town, Dubai, Hägendorf, Hong Kong, Indianapolis, Maidenhead,
Manila, New Delhi, Singapore, Sydney, Tehran, Vienna
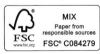 Member of the World Sport Publishers' Association (WSPA), www.w-s-p-a.org
Printed by Print Consult GmbH, Munich, Germany
Printed in Slovakia

ISBN: 978-1-78255-261-1
Email: info@m-m-sports.com
www.thesportspublisher.com

CONTENTS

INTRODUCTION

In order to understand the thought process behind *Run. Walk. Eat.*, we have to go back quite a few years, before I was a dietitian, before I was a marathoner, to 2005, when I was standing on the stage for the first time at the Walt Disney World Marathon. I googled "marathon distance" the night before the race to make sure I was understanding correctly. People were going to voluntarily wake up early in the morning to run farther than I preferred to drive. This would take hours. I was confused. This seemed like a feat reserved for the most elite athletes in the world. I didn't know what to expect. Watching my first marathon finish line changed my opinion. I saw so many victories from so many types of athletes. I got it. I wanted to run a marathon! But running the whole time seemed exhausting . . . and scary.

Luckily, I found Jeff Galloway and his run-walk-run method seemed something I could do. First you run. Then you walk. The walk breaks allowed my brain and body a moment to "breathe," to ease my fatigue both physically and mentally, and to keep going. In 2006 I finished my first marathon, and, in 2013, I finished another marathon of sorts and was a fully credentialed and licensed registered

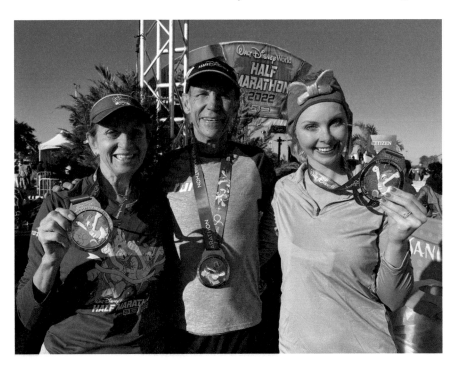

dietitian. As my studies and practical experience in dietetics grew, I saw parallels in nutrition strategies that worked and Jeff Galloway's run-walk-run strategy. Much as endlessly running seems daunting to me, for some, being expected to eat a "perfect" diet always seems equally impossible. I wondered if the "walk" break could be incorporated into the diet. The allowance of a "treat" or a small indulgence amid an otherwise nutritionally sound diet. That is where my concept for this book starts. I want to educate you on the building blocks of a balanced diet. One that not only supports weight maintenance but also includes foods that keep our bodies healthy and able to maintain our desired active lifestyle. Once you understand those concepts and have gained that education, then when you need to, you can take a "walk break" and enjoy a favorite food without the mental or physical consequences because you can use your mental tools to continue eating your well-balanced diet the rest of the time.

Run. Walk. Eat. is an education-based approach that allows you to understand food and all the good things it does for your body and your energy. You will learn the key macronutrients, micronutrients, and the portions that your body needs. You'll know the "why," and then you can learn to make better food choices a habit and not something you force yourself into. Just as I learned to enjoy long runs, you will learn to enjoy mastering your food choices and feeling better as a result of them!

Yours in good health,

Carissa Galloway

INTRODUCTION

Life Or Death—Your Diet Can Be the Difference

I had run a gentle 60-minute workout the day before and was starting the day on a rowing machine for cross training. It was a routine workout at normal exertion with no increase in huffing and puffing.

But when I stood up from the low rower seat, I was so dizzy that I had to hold on to a nearby chair—for several minutes. As I started to move toward the couch, I suddenly felt nauseous. This was a new and unsettling experience compounded by sudden extreme fatigue.

When my wife Barb returned from playing tennis an hour later, she found me on the bed, instantly knew something was wrong, and called the doctor. A series of tests ruled out most of the possible suspects, and Dr. John Marshall referred me to a cardiologist.

Because of my fitness level, even at the age of 75 and no family history of heart disease, the doctors assumed, as I did, that my heart was fine. But an echocardiogram and blood work told a different story. My right artery supplying the heart was totally blocked.

Three hours later, with five new stents, I was feeling OK. Six days later my heart failed—fortunately, a great team at the cardiac wing of Piedmont Atlanta Hospital brought me back to life.

I had averaged over an hour a day of quality exercise for over 60 years. For the previous 10 years, I had run a marathon about every month—with no issues. With no family history of heart disease and a diet very low in saturated fat, I asked the question posed by many healthy heart attack survivors: why did this happen to me?

Fortunately, my heart stoppage did not damage my brain, so I went into "investigation mode." With the help of a friend, Dave Goddard, a career journalist and investigative reporter, I found a significant cause.

During my deployment as a US Naval officer, I was stationed on a ship for 18 months that operated in coastal waters off Vietnam, where Agent Orange—a chemical herbicide and defoliant—was heavily used. Our drinking water came from the intake of sea water that was treated to remove the salt—but without any treatment or filter for this toxic carcinogen. We were drinking the chemicals and United States Department of Veterans Affairs had identified Agent Orange as a cause of heart attacks later in life.

Dr. Kohl, who conducted my stent operation brilliantly, verified that my blockage was decades old and would have normally triggered a heart attack around age 50. He said that if I had not been running for those years, I would not be alive.

Yes—regular aerobic endurance exercise has been shown to reduce heart attacks and prolong life. But I know over a dozen distance runners who died of a heart attack—and had been running more miles than I logged during the 10-year period prior to the attack—but who had unhealthy diets.

Diet Is Important!

Damaged artery walls, like mine, attract plaque that attracts cholesterol and the buildup of the products of an unhealthy diet—particularly saturated fat. This blocks the arteries.

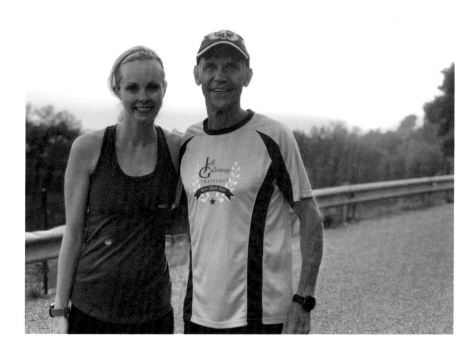

Since our marriage in 1976, Barb had cleaned up my nutrition life. For over four decades, she has provided me with mostly plant-based nutrition that included fish and chicken breast several times a month. She was saving my life before she realized that I was at risk.

In this book, Carissa not only gives you the nutrition information you need for fitness performance—but for long-term health as well. She also organizes the material for efficient access. Her explanation of the concepts is easy to understand, and the menu items offered can be acquired from a supermarket. This is truly a guidebook for your nutritional future.

It is our wish that you not just "live until you're 100," but that you run and enjoy good food until you reach that century mark.

You can do it!

Jeff Galloway

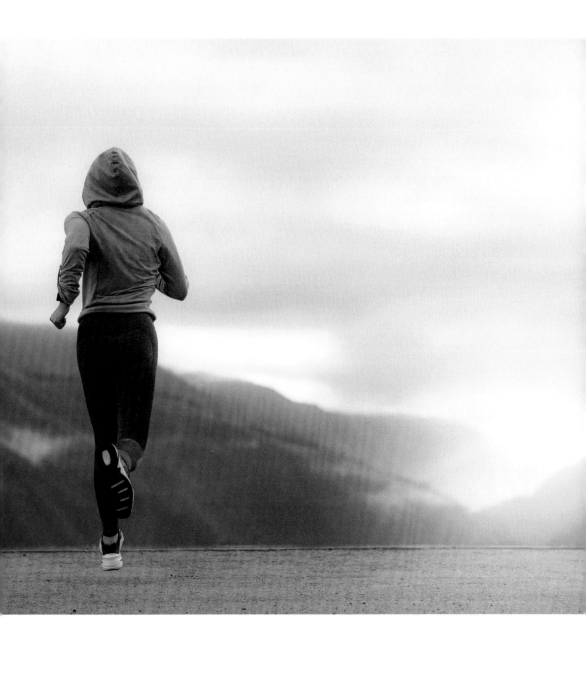

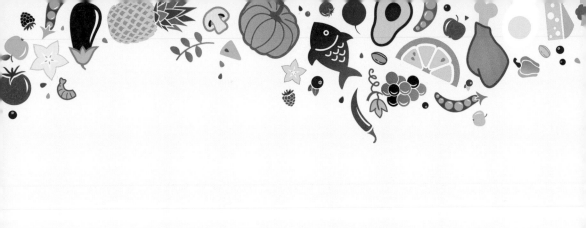

CHAPTER 1

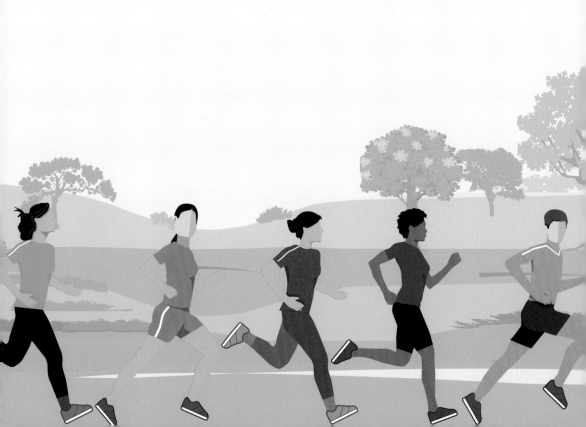

NUTRITION BASICS

You can't make better food choices if you don't understand what food is a better choice!

Carissa Galloway, RDN

How many decisions do think you make about food each day? Most people estimate about 15 when the real number is closer to 200. 200! You make 200 decisions about food each day and most of them are unconscious. Consider your morning cup of coffee—what flavor of coffee? Hot or cold? Cream or sugar? More sugar? Do I want a muffin? A second cup of coffee?

There's absolutely nothing wrong with making 200 food choices a day, however, without nutrition education you're not equipped to make the best food choices you can.

Why do these food choices matter? Good nutrition plays a role in reducing your risk of four of the top 10 leading causes of death in the US, including heart disease, cancer, stroke, and diabetes. Also if you've chosen this book, then you likely strive to lead an active lifestyle, and good nutrition will give you the energy to meet your goals and maintain an active lifestyle with all the mental and physical benefits that go along with it.

My goal for YOU is that you're informed about what to eat and what is good for your body. That's why we're starting with nutrition basics, which will help you build a better plate.

MACRONUTRIENTS

A macronutrient is a nutrient that your body needs in a large quantity to maintain the body's structure and systems. When we say "macronutrients," we are typically referring to carbohydrates, protein and fat, the nutrients we use in the largest amounts.

CARBOHYDRATES

Let's start with carbohydrates. Carbohydrates are often vilified and the first thing cut out of diets; however, carbohydrates are your body's main and preferred fuel source. According to the Dietary Guidelines for Americans (www.dietaryguidelines.gov), carbohydrates should make up 45 to 65 percent of your total daily calories. In a 2,000-calorie diet, that is roughly 900 to 1,300 calories per day from carbs. These carbohydrates are important because they give your body glucose, which then gives your body the energy to function. Glucose + energy. Your brain and blood cells rely on glucose to function, so this is a nutrient we want to build our diet around to support an active lifestyle. To further this point, the brain's only fuel is blood glucose, and if the brain doesn't get an adequate supply, it will start shutting down energy to areas that help you exercise . . . and think.

WHAT FOODS ARE CARBOHYDRATES

Carbohydrates come mainly from plant sources and include foods like:

- Grains such as breads, cereals, pasta, oatmeal, rice, crackers
- Fruits
- Beans and legumes
- Dairy products such as milk and yogurt
- Starchy vegetables such as potatoes, peas, and corn
- Sweets such as cake, cookies, candy, pies, and soda
- Juices and sports drinks
- Popcorn

Are there good carbs and bad carbs? I don't like to label foods as "good" or "bad," but from the above list, I'm sure you know some foods are more beneficial to your body than others.

When building our diet, we want to focus on the carbohydrates that contain fiber and essential vitamins, such as whole grains and beans. We also want to pick carbohydrates like fruit and vegetables because those carbohydrates are packed with vitamins, minerals, and antioxidants.

Here's an example of beneficial carbohydrates you can include in a day of eating:

- ½ cup of oatmeal cooked in 1 cup of milk with ¼ cup raspberries
- 1 apple or pear
- 1 whole wheat tortilla
- ½ cup of black beans
- 4 oz cottage cheese
- 1 small sweet potato
- 1 cup roasted broccoli.

Reducing added sugar from your diet will have a beneficial impact on your health and waistline, so limit your intake of sweets, sodas, and other high-sugar drinks. Research continues to show the dangers of too much added sugar in our diet, so let this book be your first nudge to take a close look at your diet and remove added sugars.

NATURAL VS ADDED SUGAR

Before we move onto our next macronutrient, it's important for me to reinforce the benefits of sugar from natural sources and separate them from added sugars. You have likely read a diet book or listened to a colleague on a diet tell you that they don't eat fruit because it has too much sugar. Does fruit have sugar? YES! Does this fruit sugar benefit you? YES!

The distinction is the difference between naturally occurring sugars and added sugars. Naturally occurring sugars are those found naturally in fruit and dairy foods. Added sugars are, as the name implies, sugars added to processed foods and sweets.

Naturally occurring sugars come in whole foods and are naturally packaged with other beneficial nutrients, such as fiber, vitamins, and minerals. Foods packed with fiber not only do wonders for your cholesterol and digestion but fiber

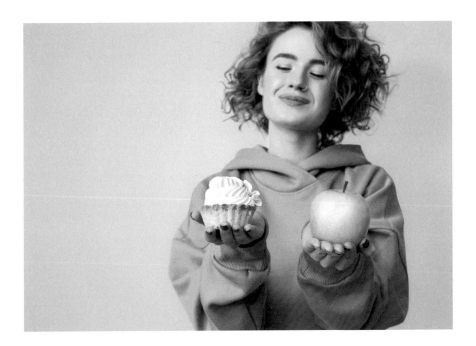

provides bulk that fills you up and makes it challenging to overeat these foods. The fiber also slows down the absorption of the naturally occurring sugar, which is beneficial to your blood sugar.

To further my point, let's compare an orange with candy orange slices:

One navel orange gives you 65 calories, over 100 percent of your daily value of vitamin C, 12 grams of naturally occurring sugar, and 3.5 grams of fiber.

Six candy orange slices give you 300 calories and 19 teaspoons of added sugar. There are no vitamins or fiber.

Which one do you think supports your overall health and active lifestyle?

If you're still unclear on added vs natural sugars, then when in doubt, read the label! Sucrose and fructose are the most common added sugars.

Added sugars can be listed on a food label in approximately 56 different varieties or names. Some of the most common include:

- Sugar
- Corn syrup or high fructose corn syrup
- Molasses
- Fructose
- Honey
- Agave syrup
- Brown rice syrup
- Cane sugar
- Corn sweetener
- Dextrose
- Evaporated cane juice
- Maltodextrin
- Xylose

The bottom line is that picking carbohydrates that are beneficial to our body can provide energy, fiber, vitamins, and minerals, and support our healthy goals.

PROTEIN

Let's look at our next beneficial macronutrient—protein. Without exaggeration, you can say that protein is the main structural and functional material in every cell in your body. Protein powers your muscles that allow you to stand, walk, run, and swim. Protein is necessary for your immune system to fight off infections. Protein allows your hair and nails to grow, and without protein you would not be able to digest the food you eat.

Protein is an essential macronutrient, and most Americans are getting adequate protein. For a 2,000 calorie-a-day diet, your recommended protein intake is between 200 and 700 calories from protein or 50 to 175 grams of protein daily.

Another way to look at it is tied to your body weight. The current RDA for protein is 0.8 grams per kilogram of body weight. Since Americans usually know their body weight in pounds and not ounces, you can use this equation to find a baseline for your protein needs:

* Multiply your weight in pounds by .36.
* For example, a person weighing 175 pounds would need at least 63 grams of protein per day.

Protein is found in many foods including:

* Meat
* Seafood
* Poultry
* Dairy Foods—milk, yogurt, cheese, cottage cheese
* Dried Beans
* Nut butters
* Nuts, seeds, and legumes
* Soy—tofu, tempeh, edamame
* Protein is also found in lower amounts in grains and some vegetables such as peas

Here's an example of protein in a day of eating that contains 72 grams of protein:

* 8 oz milk—8 grams
* 2 eggs—12 grams
* 1 tablespoon peanut butter—4 grams

- ½ cup black beans—7 grams
- 4 oz cottage cheese—14 grams
- 23 almonds—6 grams
- 3 oz salmon—21 grams

ESSENTIAL AMINO ACIDS

Protein is made up of 20 different amino acids. Nine of these are known as essential amino acids, meaning your body can't make them and you must get them from food. Eating a wide variety of foods is the best approach for meeting your protein needs. Animal proteins are the best source of essential amino acids.

We also call foods that contain all nine essential amino acids "complete protein." If you are on a vegetarian diet, you can still get all your essential amino acids. Aim to include foods like quinoa, soy/tofu, buckwheat, sprouted bread, chia seeds, spirulina, or rice and beans in your diet as often as possible.

If you are a runner or endurance athlete, you can increase your protein consumption to support your training and recovery needs. However, most research shows that endurance athletes already increase their overall caloric consumption and with this increase comes more protein. It's worth noting that your body can absorb a

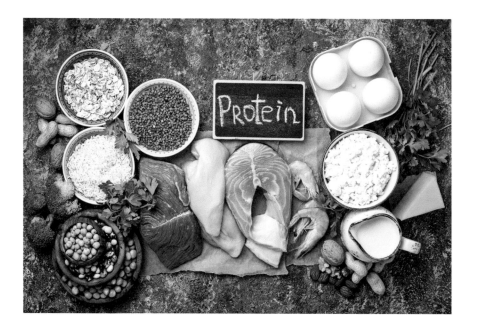

maximum of 25 grams of protein in one sitting, so make sure to space out your protein consumption throughout the day.

Finally, we need to address the dangers of eating too much protein. First, a diet that is too high in protein may increase the risk of heart disease, kidney stones, osteoporosis, and some types of cancer. A high protein intake can also replace other beneficial foods in the body. Lastly, too much protein will still be considered extra calories in the body and can be stored as fat.

FATS

Over the past 30 years, the concept of dietary fats has gone through a major transformation. Since the low-fat diets that were popular in the 1980s, we've had a nutrition education renaissance to stop our fat phobia. We now view fats as an essential part of our diet that fuels everything from satiety to giving your body energy, protecting your organs, supporting cell growth, and keeping blood pressure and cholesterol in normal levels. Yes, fats are your friend and don't necessarily make you "fat" or gain weight by eating them. Keep in mind that fats are more calorically dense than carbohydrates or protein. While carbohydrates and protein contain 4 calories per gram, fats have 9 calories per gram. This means that the calorie count can add up quickly, and you need to be more aware of portion size when you include fats in your diet.

The amount of fats you eat per day should account for 20 to 35 percent of your daily caloric intake, which is 44 to 77 grams of fat per day on a 2,000-calorie diet.

Fats can be described as "good" and "bad" depending on their molecular structure and the impact they have on your body. While I don't like to label anything in your diet as "good" or "bad," I believe the distinction here is justified.

The good fats are polyunsaturated and monounsaturated fats, and the bad fats, or those we want to limit in our diets, are trans fats and saturated fats.

THE GOOD FATS

Polyunsaturated and monounsaturated fats typically come from plant sources and are liquid at room temperature. The benefit of those unsaturated fats, according to research, is that regular consumption can reduce bad cholesterol levels in the blood, which reduces your risk of heart attack and stroke. These oils also provide vitamin E in the diet, which is an antioxidant that most Americans aren't getting enough of.

Examples of polyunsaturated and monounsaturated fats include:

- Olive oil
- Canola oil
- Sesame oil
- Avocado
- Nut butters
- Walnuts
- Soy—soybeans and tofu
- Flaxseeds
- Chia seeds

These fats are needed in our diet, and eating them regularly can support heart health. In fact, scientific evidence suggests but does not prove that eating an ounce and a half per day of most nuts as part of a diet low in saturated fat and cholesterol may reduce the risk of heart disease.

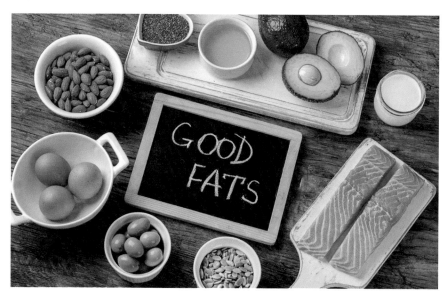

THE BAD FATS

The fats you want to limit in your diet are saturated and trans fats. These have limited if any benefits to your health and overconsumption will increase your bad cholesterol and risk of heart disease and stroke. Saturated fats are solid at room temperature and come from animal sources, full-fat dairy, eggs, and tropical oils such as coconut and palm oils. The reason most medical experts recommend a reduction in saturated fats is because these fats can increase your cholesterol, which increases your risk of heart disease and strokes.

I am well aware that there are many diets out there that include foods with saturated fats in high amounts, and I'm aware that nutrition science and "best practices" can change over time. However, it's my recommendation that to keep your heart and arteries in their best shape you should limit your intake of saturated fats. There are plenty of plant-based fats that can be a part of your diet and better support an active lifestyle.

The other fat to avoid is trans fats. Trans fats are the result of hydrogenation of an oil that allows it to provide foods with a longer shelf life and better resistance to spoiling. This is why trans fats are used in many processed goods. While saturated fats are bad for your heart, trans fats are WORSE! Not only do trans fats increase your bad or LDL cholesterol levels but they also cause a decrease in your good or HDL cholesterol levels. Trans fats are found in commercially prepared baked goods, margarines, fried foods, packaged snacks and cookies, shortening, and prepared salad dressings. Please avoid these foods as much as possible. If the food you're eating has to be unwrapped from a package, then it likely has trans fats and is a food you should try to eliminate from your diet.

I want you to take care of your body, and any food that contains an item chemically designed to prolong a shelf life doesn't have a place inside you. If you want to prolong your own shelf life, swap items with trans fats for more of a whole food or a baked good or snack that you prepared yourself.

Examples of trans and saturated fats you should AVOID include:

- Butter
- Ghee
- Coconut oil*
- Palm oil
- Lard
- Fatty cuts of meat

- Sausage
- Bacon
- Cured meats
- Full fat cheese
- Cream
- Biscuits
- Cakes
- Pies
- Cookies
- Doughnuts
- Ice cream
- Microwave popcorn
- Fried foods—French fries, chicken nuggets, fried fish
- Stick margarine
- Nondairy coffee creamer

*Coconut oil is noted because it's designation as a "bad fat" is controversial. This is because it's a saturated fat from a plant and not an animal source. It can also contain medium-chain triglycerides, which are digested by your body differently to other saturated fats.

Coconut oil, however, is NOT a super food. Scientifically, coconut oil is a saturated fat and contains even more saturated fats than butter. Increased consumption of coconut oil will raise both your bad cholesterol and your good cholesterol. Compared with other plant oils, like olive or canola, it lacks the heart health benefits of those polyunsaturated fats.

My take on coconut oil is somewhere in the middle as research is still emerging. It's neither a hero nor a villain. I don't want you to add tablespoons of it to your morning coffee, and I also don't think you have to completely omit it from your diet if it's something you enjoy cooking with. If you want to use one tablespoon two to three times a week, then go ahead, but other plant oils will give you greater benefits.

Here's an example of 55 grams GOOD-FOR-YOU fats in a day of eating:

- 2 eggs—9 grams
- 1 cup of pea milk—4.5 grams
- 23 almonds—14 grams
- ¼ avocado—5 grams
- 1 tablespoon of olive oil to cook—14 grams
- 2 tablespoons of hummus—3 grams
- 3 ounces salmon—5.5 grams.

ESSENTIAL FATTY ACIDS—OMEGA-3S

A discussion of fats would be incomplete without boosting your understanding of essential fatty acids and why we all need to strive to eat more seafood each week. Eating fats provides fatty acids that are important to your health, just like with protein. However, there are some essential fatty acids that our body can't make that we must get from food. The omega-3 fats that I'm sure you have heard so much about are essential fatty acids that we must get from our food. Failure to consume adequate amounts of these essential fatty acids can interfere with normal cell membranes, which is connected to hormone production, blood clotting, and your body's inflammatory response. A true deficiency in these essential fatty acids can even lead to the development of scaly skin! The irony of this is that omega-3s are found in fish and not having them can make your skin scaly . . . like a fish!

There is a lot of science wrapped up in omega-3s and I don't want to overwhelm you with that. Yes, there are three main omega-3 fats. Yes, omega-3s have been proven to support heart health. The strongest research has shown that omega-3s help the heart beat at a steady rhythm and keep the heart from veering into an irregular rhythm (arrythmia). Research has also shown that these cardio protective benefits of omega-3s come from eating food sources rich in omega-3s and not supplementation. Yes, I want you to eat seafood and I want you to do it at least two to three times a week.

If you take nothing else away from this book, then I hope you are inspired to eat more seafood . . . and more fiber, but we'll talk about that in a minute.

Seafood can be very easy and quick to cook. Shelf-stable canned tuna and salmon are simple ways to boost your seafood intake and take less than 10 minutes to prepare.

Easy ways to add more seafood to your diet:

- Add canned tuna or salmon to your dinner salad.
- Add tuna to cooked pasta and vegetables. Toss with Italian dressing for a tuna pasta salad.
- Order baked, boiled, or grilled fish when dining out. If you are unsure how to prepare seafood, ordering it when you dine out is a great way to experience different flavors and methods of preparation.
- Serve shrimp cocktail as a low-calorie, no-prep-required appetizer.

Recommended omega-3-rich seafood and milligrams/serving of omega-3 fatty acids:

- Farmed salmon—4,504 milligrams
- Wild salmon—1,774 milligrams
- Anchovies—1,200 milligrams
- Halibut—740 milligrams
- Albacore tuna—733 milligrams
- Mussels—665 milligrams
- Oysters—585 milligrams
- Trout—581 milligrams
- Sardines—556 milligrams
- Crab—351 milligrams
- Light tuna—228 milligrams
- Mahi Mahi—221 milligrams
- Frozen fish sticks—193 milligrams
- Lobster—71 milligrams

FIBER

Basic nutrition education is not complete without a chat about fiber. In most nutrition lectures, I talk about fiber (a lot!) because I believe it's so beneficial to your overall health and how your body feels daily. Most of us are motivated to improve our diets by the perceived benefits of the changes. Fiber has so many benefits that I think this will be one of the first nutrition upgrades you'll want to make to your current diet, and it's an easy change to make.

The benefits of fiber can include:

- Digestive support AKA "keeping us regular"
- Decreased risk of heart disease
- Helps naturally lower cholesterol
- Preliminary research supports reduction in risk of certain cancers
- Reduced risk of type II diabetes
- Blood sugar stabilization that can help control diabetes
- Reduced stress and maintaining adrenal health
- Maintaining the health of the colon
- Decreased risk of diverticulitis
- Immune health support
- Weight loss and maintenance

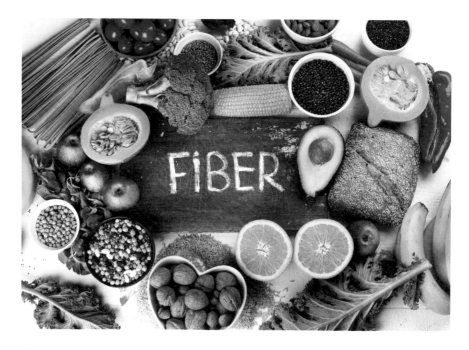

All those reasons are compelling, but I think the first one, especially for active people, is crucial. When our digestion is thrown off, we don't feel great. We can feel sluggish and bloated and that feeling of "blah" can expand into other areas of our life. On the other hand, when your digestion is working regularly, you feel light, then you have energy, and your endurance activities improve as well.

Americans spend over $700 million a year on laxative products when a boost of produce and legumes will keep them regular for much less, with the added benefits of vitamins and minerals.

HOW MUCH FIBER DO YOU NEED?

Most Americans don't get enough fiber each day. Women should try to eat at least 21 to 25 grams of fiber a day, while men should aim for 30 to 38 grams a day. One pro tip for increasing fiber . . . do it incrementally. Fiber supports your digestion, and a major increase in fiber can cause your digestion to overreact. Aim to increase your fiber intake to the recommended range over the course of 1 to 2 weeks. If you experience any gas or bloating while increasing fiber, that's a sign that what you're doing is working. Don't stop on fiber, but don't add in more until your gut flora adapts and then increase to the desired range.

Here's an example of 30 grams of fiber eaten throughout a day:

- 1 large pear with skin—7 grams
- ½ medium avocado—5 grams
- ½ cup cooked black beans—7.5 grams
- 1 cup broccoli—5 grams
- 1 cup whole wheat spaghetti—6 grams

FIBER FOR WEIGHT LOSS

If you're reading this book and weight loss is one of your goals, then you should also make increasing fiber a priority. High fiber foods, such as whole grains, fruits, vegetables, and beans, increase feelings of satiety or fullness. When you feel this satiety, you need fewer calories to feel full. When your overall caloric intake decreases, you are taking steps toward weight loss. Fiber also helps with blood sugar control, which will help prevent food cravings and allow you to make better food choices throughout the day. Finally, foods that are higher in fiber require chewing. Having to chew food, and possibly chew it longer, psychologically boosts satiety too!

MICRONUTRIENTS

We talked about macronutrients, so micronutrients need a brief introduction as well. As you can guess, the use of "micro" means we need these in smaller amounts than the macronutrients, but micronutrients are equally essential to your body. These are the vitamins and minerals that our body can't make and we must obtain from food.

Micronutrients are vitamins and minerals, and in general, they help with your well-being, your development, and disease prevention. All the micronutrients, except vitamin D, cannot be made in the body and, as such, must be taken in via diet.

The recommended amounts of micronutrients are small; however, the impact of a deficiency can be significant, so make sure they're a part of your well-balanced diet.

Some of the essential micronutrients include vitamin D, vitamin A, iron, iodine, folate, and zinc.

Do I want you to be obsessed with micronutrients? NO! This isn't a nutrition textbook, but I want you to be aware that vitamins and minerals matter. If you adopt the overall healthy eating pattern outlined in this book, then you are on your way to consuming a well-rounded diet with an emphasis on plants.

WHAT'S THE BEST DIET?

Now that you have the nutrition basics outlined, the next question is what's the BEST diet?

The good news is I have a simple answer from my years as a registered dietitian.

The best diet is . . . THE ONE YOU STICK WITH!

A meal plan for the "best diet in the world" does not benefit you if you don't stick with it! We've all tried restrictive diets, whether keto, low fat, or the carrot and hazelnut diet, followed by my co-author Jeff Galloway in the 1970s. Most of us aren't still on those diets because they weren't sustainable long term.

A well-balanced diet that incorporates whole grains, fruits, vegetables, good-for-you fats, protein, with an emphasis on fish, and fiber is the diet I want you to be on for the rest of your life. It's a diet designed by you based on your tastes and preferences. It allows for occasional treats, and it not only supports a healthy weight but your overall health too. Using the meal plans outlined later in this book, you can pick and choose meals and ideas that work for you and shape them into your ideal diet. This diet will nourish you and release you from the stress of constantly dieting or wondering if what you're eating is good for you.

If you stop me on the street and say, "Carissa, what diet should I eat for the rest of my life?" and I don't have time for the full nutrition education you're getting in this book, then I would say the Mediterranean diet. Both Jeff and I follow a diet based on the Mediterranean diet.

The Mediterranean diet is consistently ranked near the top of the world's best diets. Some of the reasons why include:

- Balance of nutrients that's nutritionally sound
- Easy to follow
- Health benefits including weight loss, heart and brain health, cancer prevention, and diabetes prevention and control.

If you're familiar with the food pyramid some of us will be familiar with from our youth, then you can look at the Mediterranean diet as having a pyramid too. What I love is that the base or bottom of the pyramid is not food at all. The base of the pyramid are the goals of being physically active and enjoying meals with others. If you're reading this book, then I know you aim to be physically active, and most humans enjoy dining with others when possible.

The pyramid continues with the bulk of your daily diet coming from fruits, vegetables, grains, olive oil, beans, nuts, legumes, seeds, herbs, and spices. Protein is the next level in a lesser amount. Fish and poultry are recommended in the Mediterranean diet with fish being consumed in greater levels than poultry.

On the same upper level as poultry are cheese, eggs, and yogurt. These can be included and enjoyed in your diet but in moderation. Wine also falls into this category as something you can enjoy in moderation.

At the top of the pyramid are other meats and sweets, and your goal is to decrease your consumption of both of these.

The Mediterranean diet is flavorful, colorful, diverse, and delicious and a great place to start upgrading your nutrition as you continue with this book.

GOOD BLOOD SUGAR = MOTIVATION

Jeff Galloway

Your brain is fueled by blood sugar. When the blood sugar level (BSL) is at a good, moderate, "normal" level you feel good, stable, and motivated. The brain monitors BSL very carefully, and if the BSL is lowered or interrupted, it will start shutting things down and triggering anxiety and negative attitude hormones.

If you are sugar sensitive and consume too much sugar, 45 or more minutes before you exercise, your BSL can rise too high. You'll feel really good for a short period, but the excess sugar triggers a release of insulin. This reduces BSL to an uncomfortable level. In this state, your energy drops, mental focus is foggy, and motivation goes down rapidly.

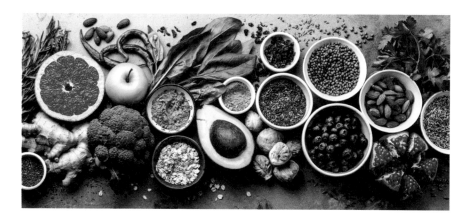

When BSL is maintained throughout the day, you will be more motivated to exercise, add other movement to your life, be mentally active, deal with stress, and solve problems. Just as eating throughout the day keeps metabolism up, the steady infusion of balanced nutrients all day long will maintain a stable BSL. This produces a feeling of well-being.

You don't want to get on the "bad side" of your BSL. Low levels are a stress on the brain—literally messing with your mind. If you have not eaten for several hours before a run or walk and your BSL drops, you'll receive an increase in the number of negative and anxiety hormones, reducing motivation to exercise.

The simple act of eating about 100 calories within 30 minutes before running can reduce the negative, make you feel good, and get you out the door. This can be the difference between whether you run, or not. The standard recommendation for all sports is 2 calories per pound of body weight. This may be too much for many runners, so you can experiment to find what works for you.

THE BSL ROLLER COASTER

Eating a snack with too many calories from simple carbohydrates can be counterproductive for BSL maintenance. As mentioned previously, when the sugar level gets too high, your body produces insulin, sending BSL lower than before. The tendency is to eat again, which produces excess calories that are converted into fat. But if you don't eat, you'll stay hungry and pretty miserable—in no mood to exercise, move around and burn calories, or get in your workout for the day. A simple solution is to eat grains instead of simple sugars or combine protein with carbs.

TRY EATING EVERY 2 TO 3 HOURS

Once it is established which snacks work best to maintain your BSL, most runners maintain a stable BSL by eating small meals regularly, every 2 to 3 hours. Overall, it's best to combine complex carbs with protein and a small amount of fat.

DO I HAVE TO EAT BEFORE RUNNING?

Only if your blood sugar is low. Most people who run in the morning don't need to eat anything before they start. But some very active people, or those who did not eat much during the evening, can experience a blood sugar drop overnight and will feel/exercise better with a pre-run snack.

As mentioned, if your BSL is low in the afternoon and you have a workout scheduled, a snack can help when taken about 30 minutes before the run. If you feel that a morning snack will help, the only issue to avoid is consuming so much that you get an upset stomach.

For best results in raising blood sugar when it is too low (within 30 minutes before a run), a snack should have about 80 percent of the calories in simple carbohydrate and 20 percent in protein. (See *Hardwired for Fitness* by Portman and Ivy) As noted when researching this book, Portman and Ivy note that the addition of 20 percent protein promotes the production of insulin, which is helpful before a run in getting the glycogen into your muscles and ready for use. If you eat an energy bar or similar snack, be sure to drink 4 to 6 ounces (120 to 180 milliliters) of water with it.

EATING DURING EXERCISE

Most exercisers don't need to worry about eating or drinking during a run until the length exceeds 90 minutes, as long as the pre-exercise fuel was at adequate levels. So when starting a run that is an hour and a half long, or longer, consume about 30 to 40 calories every 2 miles. Adjust the amount depending upon your individual needs.

The brain's fuel is blood glucose. If you don't keep this boosted during a long workout, the brain will be deprived and will start shutting things down. Avoid this by trying different snacks and using the one that works best for you.

JEFF'S Rule of Thumb: 30 to 40 calories about every 2 miles (20 to 30 minutes), with 2 to 4 ounces of water (60 to 120 milliliters).

Easiest to digest:

- Candy—particularly gummi bears or hard candies, such as lifesavers.
- Sugar Cubes or tablets—This is the simplest of the BSL booster snacks and the easiest on the stomach for most runners.

Other products:

- Energy Bars—Cut into small pieces. Avoid products with a lot of fiber, fat, or protein.
- Gel products—these come in small packets and are the consistency of honey or thick syrup. The most successful way to take them is to put one to three packets in a small plastic bottle with a pop-top. About every 10 to 15 minutes, take a small amount with a sip or two of water. CAUTION: Many runners report nausea at the end of races when using this type of product.
- Sports Drinks—I've noticed that a significant percentage of my runners who drink sports drinks during a run experience nausea. If you have found this to work for you, use it exactly as you have used it before. During a run, I recommend water.

IT IS IMPORTANT TO RELOAD WITHIN 30 MINUTES AFTER EXERCISE

Whenever you have finished a hard or long workout (for you), a recovery snack can help you recover faster. Again, the 80/20 ratio of simple carbohydrate to protein has been most successful in reloading the muscles.

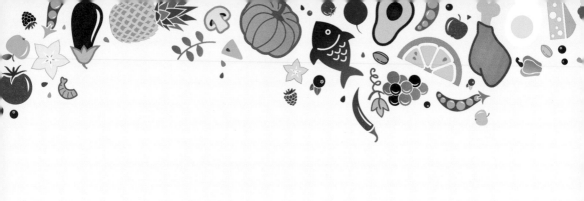

CHAPTER 2

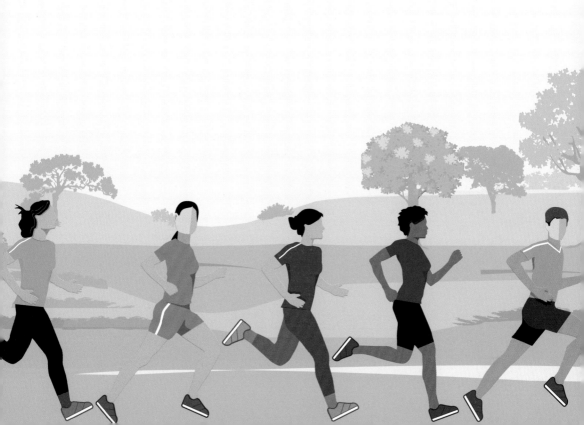

BEFORE CHOOSING YOUR FOOD, CHOOSE THE BEST BRAIN TO MANAGE HUNGER, CRAVINGS, ENERGY, FATIGUE, AND FAT

Jeff Galloway

You have two brains that control eating—and YOU can choose which one will take control:

1. The Ancient Subconscious-Reflex Brain (SB), which will trigger mindless, unaccountable eating
2. The Human-Conscious Brain (CB), which can give you control over quality, quantity, and weight control
3. Using cognitive strategies can help you make the changes you desire:
   • Avoid mindless eating by managing nutrition
   • Ensure you're getting adequate nutrients
   • Enjoy food without adding extra calories
   • Change begins with a strategy and focusing on each food item you eat
   • Healthy food can taste as good as junk food.

Over half of the population is significantly overweight or obese, and I communicate with many of these citizens every week. Most want to change eating habits and exercise more but say they are too busy. So they allow the SB to choose foods that taste good—without accountability.

This ancient brain (SB) has reflex-eating circuits that are millions of years old and are designed to avoid starvation—which our ancient ancestors faced constantly. These circuits stimulate overeating when food is available due to a series of digestive secretions. For example, eating foods that have sugar, salt, and fat will trigger the release of dopamine—"the joy hormone." Eat a potato chip and you get a jolt of dopamine pleasure. When you give control to the subconscious brain, the next action is a reflex—to reach for another chip, and then another. There's no accountability when the ancient brain is in control.

The strategies in this book work because they activate the human brain (CB), which overrides the SB and gives you control. You can then set up strategies and focus on food and exercise choices. You now have the ability to make changes in your nutrition, improve vitality, and enhance the quality of your life.

You'll learn about many successful strategies from Carissa, such as using a nutrition app. As you interact with your app to choose foods and track nutrition and calories, you become accountable and can achieve your nutrition goals.

It's not really about discipline and dedication but about mentally focusing on the enrichment and pleasure that exercise brings to your life. You need the calories that good snacks provide to sustain energy all day long—and to fuel the muscles during exercise. As you focus on the reasons for choosing each food, you put your CB in control.

Each of us is capable of using our human CB to control our nutrition and get motivated to start and continue exercising. In the process, we can find far more joy throughout the mind-body network from making healthy food choices and exercising than we did from eating potato chips and bonbons while sitting on the couch.

SERIOUS RUNNERS ALSO BENEFIT

Many talented and dedicated runners tell me that they tried to eat better but relapsed back into the "comfort foods" containing sugar salt and fat—often rationalizing that they need the calories to fuel their strenuous exercise. The reality is that giving the reflex brain permission to eat junk often leads to consuming more calories than they are burning. So they ask, "How can I train for a half/full marathon and gain weight?"

At the same time, junk food won't provide the nutrients needed for repair and performance. After 4 to 6 months under the reflex brain "dopamine diet," I receive confessions that nutrition might be responsible for the "lingering fatigue" and lower quality in their workouts and races.

Nutrition is only one piece of the performance puzzle. But if you don't get the quality fuel to do the workouts and rebuild afterward, training will suffer and later, race performance.

A few key nutritional "edits" can be a significant mental catalyst during the improvement journey. If you are making good food choices and monitoring this, you'll be more positive about the ability to perform workouts on a tough day. You'll gain confidence in your diet and training and will likely feel better, with more energy.

The simple strategies in this book make you the "captain of your nutrition ship." Just as my training methods activate your human brain to control the training process, you'll learn how to set up a cognitive eating plan and keep it on track. Not only can this give you the edge on recovery and sustained energy as the training improves but you will improve health and overall well-being. When you combine enjoyable aerobic running with a mental focus on eating, you can feel better, perform better, recover faster, reduce general fatigue, and burn more fat—for a better life.

But we have many subconscious eating patterns that are deeply embedded in our SB brain. In this chapter I will tell you about the exciting research showing how you can consciously activate CB circuits to give you control over subconscious eating patterns that lower our energy and reduce motivation for running.

We have a powerful mind-body network that is interconnected. Eating influences mental activity, and mental activity influences eating—all day long.

Yes, you can harness this network to be the master of your nutrition, feel better, and improve health while controlling diet/weight and performance nutrition.

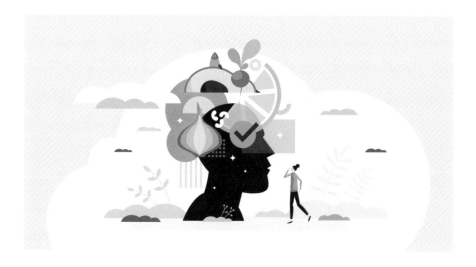

WHO'S IN CHARGE: CONSCIOUS BRAIN OR SUBCONSCIOUS REFLEX BRAIN?

At any given moment, you can choose one of two brain operating systems: 1) The more ancient SB located in the brainstem, or 2) the human CB located in the frontal lobe.

The challenge: SB gratification eating patterns. Most humans, most of the time, allow the subconscious "reflex" brain to choose what and when to eat. This is natural because the SB conducts most of our activities throughout the day. Hardwired in this ancient and continuously upgraded brainstem are thousands of genetically embedded and learned behavior patterns that evolved millions of years ago in response to the constant threat of starvation. To enhance survival, our SB developed many circuits that stimulate us to eat whenever food is available and make us feel good when we EAT sugar and fat. Brain circuits keep rewarding us with the "joy" hormone dopamine even when we've eaten far more than we need for the next day or two without feeling satisfied.

Overeating can compromise goals even for skinny runners. Even if you don't need or want to lose weight, subconscious eating patterns can cause gastrointestinal issues that may keep you from your goals. The simple cognitive eating plans in this book can help you make the best choices before and after workouts and races so you can perform at your best.

USE YOUR CB AND GAIN CONTROL OVER EATING

You can take control of your nutritional destiny by having a cognitive strategy for eating (or any other activity). This shifts control out of the SB and into the CB. As you focus on what you eat, how much, when, etc., the CB overrides the SB. This interrupts embedded emotional subconscious eating patterns and gives you a chance to choose foods that will keep you energized and healthy while you avoid overeating. By having an eating plan, you can combine the foods you need to balance your nutrients, keep the energy supply flowing, and avoid dehydration. By using the right combination of seasonings, healthy food can taste great!

You don't have to give up the foods you love, but for nutritional success, you need a strategy and a plan. As you interact with this plan throughout the day, you turn on the CB and gain control.

HOW SB CIRCUITS WORK

1. SB circuits are set up to eat when food is available. Most of the energy and eating circuits were developed over millions of years when food was scarce, and starvation was common. For survival, our appetite circuit is turned on when food is available and is not turned off until we have eaten far more than we need for that day and often the next day or two. The extra volume is more likely to provide the individual with the vitamins, minerals, protein, etc., to repair bio damage and keep the body running.

2. Subconscious dopamine reflex eating—no accountability. Many of the subconscious reflex brain eating patterns are not healthy or beneficial for running. Take the dopamine reflex reward pattern, for example. Dopamine is a neurotransmitter—a hormone that delivers a more powerful sense of joy than most. When you eat a food with sugar, salt, and/or fat, such as a potato chip (which has all three), you get a good dose of dopamine, which feels so good and is gone so fast that you reach for another, and then another. If you choose to stay under the control of the SB, there is no accountability as you pile on the calories. Such eating patterns produced greater fat storage in our ancestors, which gave them a chance to make it through the weeks when food was not available.

3. Stress stimulates subconscious eating patterns. The SB, when we allow it to be in control, will monitor overall stress. As stress levels increase to (what it determines to be) overload, the SB will trigger the release of anxiety and negative attitude hormones. One of the most common circuits activated to counter this stress/negative attitude buildup is the dopamine reflex. The simple subconscious fix to the release of negative attitude hormones triggered by stress, developed over millions of years is to reach for sugar/salt/fat and feel better quick (but only temporarily). Many runners justify "carbohydrate loading" by SB snacking to counter the stress of an upcoming race or long run—and then run the race carrying a pound or more of carbohydrate-loading baggage.

So it is common, when stressed or very tired, to subconsciously reach for sugar/salt/fat snacks to get a dose of dopamine. Unfortunately, the reward is very temporary and then requires multiple doses with no accountability. Again, the way you can gain control is to have a strategy in place.

Damage from addictive eating patterns. Dr. Pam Peeke, in her book *The Hunger Fix,* has noted research showing how addictive eating patterns can damage the natural reward centers of the brain so that more and more junk food is needed for gratification. Ultimately there is no satisfaction and less and less dopamine when large amounts are ingested. She has also identified a "detox program" with exercise and eating plans that have helped thousands to enjoy eating healthy food. Here are some of the many insightful tips from this book.

- A diet full of unhealthy fat, salt, and sugar switches on certain genes to cope.
- As one savors sugar, histones direct genes to increase insulin.
- Increased insulin, with excess unhealthy sugar calorie intake, increases fat storage.
- Regular, repeated ingestions/insulin secretions, CAN result in insulin resistance and type 2 diabetes.
- Too much food intake stimulates creation of fat cells.
- Higher levels of fat trigger hormones that increase pain in joints and "weak links."

ENERGY IS THE FIRST PRIORITY

Forward movement kept our ancient ancestors alive: the more territory covered, the more food-gathering possibilities. Maintaining energy is top priority throughout the mind-body network, and there are many effective brain circuits that keep the energy flowing even when there are challenges.

The brain's only fuel is blood glucose. When the supply of blood sugar is adequate, the brain will keep the many complex systems going, including an adequate energy system for the muscles to do their work. If we don't eat regularly and there is an interruption/lowering of the BSL, the brain will start reducing blood flow to key areas, lowering the metabolism/energy level, reducing brain function, and shutting systems down.

FAT IS THE BACKUP FUEL

We are hardwired to store fat for survival. Numerous internal circuits connect mind and body to ensure energy supply when food supply is below current energy needs or unavailable (periods of starvation). The brain circuit, commonly called the "set point," maintains and monitors fat storage and triggers an increase in appetite when the set point is low and food is available. When on a dramatic calorie reduction, fat is released. The set point has memory, however. When one has lost 30 pounds due to a continued starvation diet, for example, and returns to eating "normal levels," the set point stimulates hunger a bit more, day after day, until the (pre-diet) set point of fat is reached—often with additional pounds around the waistline.

- Your energy supply system is designed to adapt to regular aerobic exercise. Exercising about every other day will keep these circuits in good operation, while the CB searches for more efficient ways of eating, repairing, storing, and burning.
- In most workouts, intensity should be low for fat burning and appetite management. Workouts need to be "aerobic," meaning "no huffing and puffing."
- Use my run-walk-run method! By adjusting the amounts of running and walking, you can reduce the intensity and stress—staying in the aerobic zone.
- Gentle aerobic running stimulates production of BDNF—miracle grow for the brain and nerves, also important for memory, learning, critical thinking. and decision making.
- The meditative effect of a gentle run/walk can help in the healing of dopamine damage from addictive eating patterns. (Dr. Peeke)
- Anaerobic exercise (working hard so that you are huffing and puffing) doesn't burn fat, shuts down digestive blood flow, reduces ability to reload within 30 minutes, and stimulates hunger. If you want to improve your race times, some anaerobic workouts are necessary—but only one to two per week.
- Once you burn a threshold of calories each day (usually 700 to 900 calories) the appetite circuit tends to curb hunger.

THE SATISFACTION CIRCUIT

The hunger reduction brain circuit is turned on by reaching a threshold of calories burned each day. The amount needed is between 700 and 900 calories from all sources, according to Portman and Ivy in *Hardwired for Fitness.* So for those wanting to lose weight/burn fat, gentle exercise in the morning can give one a head start on managing appetite for the rest of the day.

THE GOOD ATTITUDE CIRCUIT

It is well established that running activates your "good attitude" better than just about anything you can do. Run gently, turn on a good attitude, and you will be less susceptible to dopamine eating.

THE VITALITY CIRCUIT

Thousands of runners have reported experiences similar to what happened to me recently. Arriving home after a long day, I felt too tired with no energy to exercise. The run was scheduled but there seemed to be no resources to run for a minute or two—30 minutes seemed impossible. Promising myself that I would only go for 5 minutes, I got out the door. Surprisingly, the energy started flowing. Day after day I have found that after 5 minutes (using the right run-walk-run strategy for the day), I keep going past 10, 20, 30 minutes with no problems. I had more energy afterward to work on projects all evening. Running at the right pace from the beginning (with the right ratio of walk breaks) activates the vitality circuit. This often reduces the craving and intake of snacks normally needed to boost blood sugar on a stressful day.

THE EMPOWERMENT CIRCUIT

Finishing a run, especially on a tough day, turns on the empowerment circuit, which can give you the mental control to take care of your eating and your life. Running tends to activate the CB, which overrides the SB. When running regularly, runners tell me that they feel more motivated to change their diet for the better. This is backed by research.

TOOLS THAT GIVE YOU CONTROL OVER NUTRITION

As noted, most humans allow the emotional SB circuits to guide our eating behaviors, craving sugary/salty/fatty foods for the temporary good feelings of a dopamine release. Other subconscious circuits are triggered to continue eating well past nutritional needs to store fat.

You can choose the circuits in your brain that you want to use every time you decide to eat something. "Deciding" will activate the CB. If you have a cognitive eating strategy, you can control what goes in your mouth, maintain energy and BSL, balance nutritional elements, and avoid a fat increase. This is frontal lobe eating with accountability. You are in charge!

You don't have to eat a large quantity of food to get the right balance of nutrients—you simply need to engage your CB and do the accounting.

1. Write everything down that you eat: food, amount (ingredients if in a product).
2. Enter your data into a website, app or a journal.
3. Analyze your results every day or two.

All these activate the human CB so that you are in control. As you do this regularly, you will shift to CB control as you consider something to eat. Most runners who have done this tell me they have progressively chosen healthier choices and reduced the "dopamine junk" choices.

By using the CB, you can set up an eating strategy, monitor intake, ensure adequate consumption of vitamins/minerals/protein, and gain control over your eating. In this book you will learn the key principles in each area with cognitive strategies. This means that you can focus on each issue several times a day and set up your plan to stay on track.

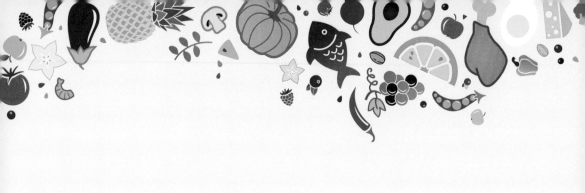

CHAPTER 3

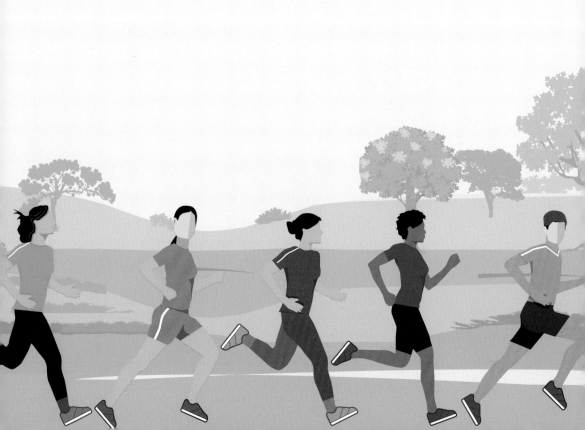

NUTRITION AND RUNNING (OR TRAINING)

When you go the distance, you have to fuel your body to do the same! Learn the nutrition your body needs for training.

Carissa Galloway, RDN

NUTRITION FOR TRAINING

One of the standard lines in my sports nutrition seminar is, "I don't care if you run a 5-minute mile or a 15-minute mile . . . if you're going the distance, you're an athlete, and you need to fuel like one!"

As you increase your runs, cycling miles, or exercise, your body adapts. It needs more fuel (carbohydrates), it needs more raw building materials to strengthen your muscles (protein), and it needs more support to keep you healthy (antioxidants). Training, at its core, breaks down your body. The goal is to break down your body to build you up to be stronger in both endurance and strength. However, your body can't rebuild without having the essential nutrition for an athlete. In this chapter, you'll learn how to give your body what it needs so you can sustain your active lifestyle.

 LET'S TALK HYDRATION

HOW DO YOU GET THE ENERGY FOR EXERCISE?

The magic word for you having the energy to complete a sustained workout is GLYCOGEN! During exercise, you get energy from carbohydrates via the glucose in your blood stream and from stored glycogen in your muscles and liver.

When you start a long workout, your body is conveniently carrying glycogen for you. The total amount of energy stored as carbohydrate in the body is about 2,600 calories and of that about 2,000 can be used. This is enough energy to sustain you for about 2 hours of continuous exercise.

The takeaway point from this is two-fold. First, as you just read, you have enough stored energy for about 2 hours of exercise. Therefore, you mainly need to fuel during prolonged exercise. Second, as an athlete, you need to refill your glycogen stores continually. When your muscles are depleted of glycogen, you experience fatigue and your performance decreases.

If you're wondering if you can have 4,000 calories of pizza and waffles after your long run and give your glycogen stores an extra boost for the next run, then I'm going to have to burst your bubble. Your body has a finite ability to store carbohydrates in your muscle and liver. Once those stores are filled, you will store extra excess glucose as added fat. Therefore, it's important to maintain a balanced diet with carbohydrates, but not overeat or overfuel after runs to maintain a healthy weight.

You do have one way to boost the glycogen stores in your muscles outside of food. That is commitment to proper training. Research has shown that well-trained muscles may be able to hold 20 to 50 percent more glycogen than untrained muscles. This means that well-conditioned muscles can sustain endurance exercise longer, and you can further support that by combining the correct amount of carbohydrates in your diet and following a training plan.

It's important to note that the intensity of your exercise will determine the amount of carbohydrates used. You will not use the same amount of glycogen for a leisurely walk as you would running a 10k race, even if you were moving for the same amount of time.

WHAT ABOUT USING FAT FOR ENERGY?

Your body does use fat for energy. In fact, for low-to-moderate intensity activities, fat will provide nearly all your energy needs. Using fat for energy requires more oxygen, which is why it's possible for low-intensity exercise, but not for more vigorous intensity workouts.

Just like trained muscles can hold more glycogen, endurance training boosts your body's cardiovascular capabilities and thus increases your body's utilization of fat for energy. This also "saves" your muscle glycogen stores for later use. Look at all the benefits of living an active lifestyle!

WHAT ABOUT CARB LOADING?

Jeff is going to share his thoughts from his 60+ years of experience fueling for long runs later in this chapter, but carb loading is a concept that I'm frequently asked about as a runner and dietitian. When I'm talking to an elite athlete, I highly recommend a strict, typical 7-day carb-loading protocol. With everyday athletes or those who are training for races but are also on a weight-loss journey, the answer is more complicated.

Do you need more carbohydrates to perform at your best in runs of over 90 minutes? Yes!

Will an extra-large pasta dinner the night before a race or long run improve your performance? No! And it might make you feel bloated and sluggish.

WHAT IS A TRADITIONAL CARBOHYDRATE-LOADING PLAN?

The goal of carb loading before an endurance event is to maximize the storage capacity of your muscle glycogen. Just like putting gas into your car before a long drive, carb-loading puts more fuel into your muscles for your upcoming endurance event. Not everyone will have improved performance from carb loading. In fact, research has shown that women are less likely to have improved performance from carb loading. This is because women oxidize more fat and less carbohydrate and protein than men during endurance exercise. (I told you this was complicated!)

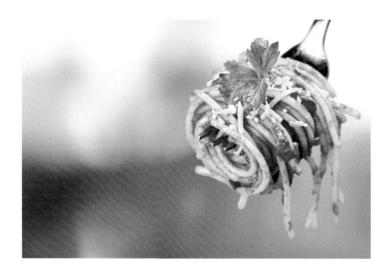

TRADITIONAL CARB-LOADING REGIMEN

I do not recommend a traditional carb-loading regimen for most people. I am sharing it here to enhance your knowledge, but know for the general public that I recommend the modified carb loading detailed in the next section.

The traditional carb-loading regimen starts about 7 days before your endurance event. Carbs are an important part of this process, but they're not everything. Remember how you're eating carbs to fill up your glycogen stores? With this in mind, logically you need to limit activity to prevent using up those glycogen stores.

The first part of traditional carb loading is to taper exercise by doing a little less each day in the 7 days leading up to an endurance event. Many people find this hard mentally, but this is necessary to preserve muscle glycogen, and it's recommended in both this traditional carb-loading regimen and the modified version. The second part of carb loading is an increased carbohydrate consumption. The following schedule is one that is recommended for elite athletes. It's advised to increase carbohydrate consumption based on the following schedule:

- Days 4 to 6 prior to your endurance event, 4 to 5 grams of carbohydrates per kilogram* of body weight each day.
- Days 1 to 3 prior to your endurance event, 8 to 10 grams of carbohydrates per kilogram of body weight each day.
- About 3 hours before the event, eat 200 to 300 grams of carbohydrate.

*NOTE: To find your body weight in kilograms, divide your weight in pounds by 2.2.

To make this balance of calories work, you will be reducing your intake of both protein and fat to account for the extra calories from carbohydrates. If you do the math, 10 grams of carbohydrates per kilogram of body weight each day is A LOT! For a 175-pound person that is about 795 grams of carbs per day, which equates to 3,100 calories from carbs. That's a lot of carbs, but still, this is a protocol I recommend for an elite athlete. However, I do not recommend this for someone running for fun or to enjoy the benefits of exercise or a race with friends; it's simply too many calories and that high caloric intake can be hard to achieve without the constant supervision of a dietitian. The reason this is explained here is because I wanted you to see the traditional protocol. Should you choose to enter a strict training regimen for a personal best, this could be something you consider. For other long runs, my expert opinion is that it's too many calories and, in most everyday athletes, the benefit to exercise doesn't outweigh the risk of all the excess calories and diversion from an individual's standard diet. My preferred carb-loading system for non-elite athletes is outlined next.

MODIFIED CARB-LOADING REGIMEN

For most adults striving for an active lifestyle by running and training for endurance events, I recommend a modified carb-loading regimen before your long runs or endurance events. This will give you the adequate fuel for long events, but it will prevent overeating and "rationalizing" the necessary extreme levels of carbohydrates and calories that could lead to weight gain.

In the modified carb-loading regimen, I recommend that you add in one additional carb in the 5 days leading up to the race. Have two pieces of bread, eat the whole potato, or have pasta and a slice of garlic bread.

The morning of the race, eat 150 to 200 grams of carbohydrates 3 to 4 hours before the race. One hour before the event, have a small carbohydrate snack, like a small banana, some dry cereal, or sports drink. Also make sure you're consuming water before your event. The suggested ratio is 5 to 7 milliliters of water per kilogram of bodyweight.

If you weigh 175 pounds, divide your weight by 2.2 to get your weight in kilograms. For someone who weighs 175 pounds, that would be 79. 5 kilograms. Your fluid range would be 398 to 556 milliliters. That translates to 13 to 18 ounces of fluid. Do this in the hours leading up to exercise so you have time to hydrate and use the restroom before your event or long run starts!

This pre-event formula of a carb heavy meal and hydration should not be tried just on race morning. Nothing new on race morning! You should practice this formula and routine with every run or endurance event over 90 minutes.

The final takeaway on carb loading is that physiologically you need to increase carbohydrate consumption before endurance activities over 90 minutes to keep your glycogen stores full to provide you with the energy for exercise. This is best done in the days before your endurance event and not the night before. For everyday athletes, this can be done by a small increase in total caloric intake, a shift to more carbohydrates, and a reduced intake of protein and fats.

 MORE ON FUELING FOR THE LONG RUN

PROTEIN AND ENDURANCE EXERCISE

If carbohydrates are the key to energy before exercise, then protein is the key to recovery after. Protein literally provides your body with the building blocks to get stronger, faster, and to prevent injury.

The primary function of protein is to build and maintain tissues. Protein is also the basis of enzymes, hormones, and the immune system proteins.

Do you need more protein as an athlete? Yes, but maybe no. The amount of protein recommended for athletes is usually higher than nonathletes. However, protein consumption in most of our standard diets usually exceeds recommendations for both nonathletes and athletes. As you achieve your goals for an active lifestyle, you may find that you don't need to add more protein to your diet, rather you need to focus on the timing of the protein to get maximum benefits.

The Dietary Reference Intake for adults is 0.8 grams of protein per kilogram of body weight daily. For endurance athletes this can go up to 1.2 to 1.4 grams of protein per kilogram of body weight daily.

When you exercise, you put your body into a catabolic state. Catabolic means that you have broken down tissues to give yourself the energy to sustain the exercise. You break down carbohydrates, fats, and protein, and that's okay! However, in order to rebuild and reverse the catabolic state, you need to consume both protein and carbohydrates following exercise. The best time to do this is 1 to 2 hours after exercise.

PRE-WORKOUT MEAL IDEAS

During pre-workout, the focus is on carbohydrates with minimal fat and fiber. Add in a little protein to boost satiety if you can tolerate that. These higher calorie meals should be eaten 1 to 2 hours before exercise. Some examples include:

- Ricotta cheese on cinnamon raisin toast
  - » ⅓ cup of part skimmed ricotta cheese on one to two slices of whole grain cinnamon raisin toast
- Peanut butter toast
  - » 1 to 2 teaspoons natural peanut butter on two slices of Ezekiel bread or whole wheat English muffin

- Instant oatmeal with banana slices
- Fruit smoothie made with Greek yogurt
- Granola bar or belVita crackers
- 10 whole grain crackers with two slices of low-sodium deli meat
- 1 cup low-fat cottage cheese with ½ cup fresh berries
- ½ cup spaghetti with marinara sauce

If you are only 30 minutes away from exercise, try these pre-workout snack ideas. Also include 5 to 10 ounces of water to keep you hydrated before exercise.

- Medium piece of fresh fruit—banana, orange, pear
- 1 sports GU/gel
- 4 to 6 ounces of sports drink
- 3 pitted dates
- Rice cake
- Applesauce pouch
- ½ cup of dry cereal, such as Cheerios

POST-WORKOUT MEAL IDEAS

Your post-workout meal can be something like a protein smoothie, or it can be a normal meal. When I work with runners or other athletes, I'm often surprised at the "narrow" view of the post-workout meal that has developed. People tend to think of post-workout eats as only protein shakes or bars. The truth is that you're looking for the correct

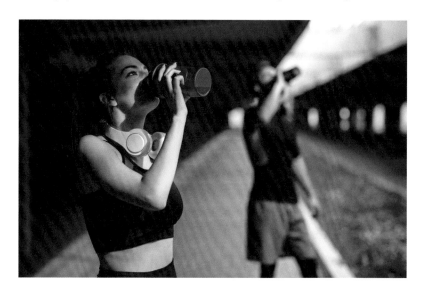

macronutrients, and that's it. These can be in a shake or the lunch you have every day. What you choose to eat really depends on your schedule, however, the key is to not go over 60 minutes without getting protein and carbohydrates into your body to start the recovery process. You can also eat a normal meal after exercise. Just because it's "post exercise" doesn't mean it has to be a meal that's thought of post workout. It can be, but the key is the carbohydrate and protein. Those building blocks jump start your recovery whether they're from a perfectly designed smoothie or leftover fried rice.

POST-WORKOUT SNACK IDEAS

- 8 ounces low-fat chocolate milk
- Ready-to-drink protein shake with a piece of fruit
- 1 slice of whole wheat toast with nut butter and sliced strawberries
- 2 graham crackers with nut butter and 12 blueberries
- 1 to 2 hard-boiled eggs with 8 whole wheat crackers.

POST-WORKOUT MEAL IDEAS

- Burrito bowl
  - » ¾ cup brown rice, ½ cup black beans, 4 ounces chicken, fajita veggies, salsa, guacamole
- Protein bento box, such as from Starbucks
  - » Hard-boiled egg, edamame, hummus, whole wheat crackers, cheese stick, dried fruit
- Spaghetti
  - » 4 ounces ground turkey with ¾ cup whole wheat spaghetti and marinara sauce
- 6-inch tuna salad sub on whole wheat with veggies
- 3 egg veggie omelet with roasted potatoes
- Hashbrown egg nests (recipe in book)
- Mediterranean Hash (recipe in book)
- Tart Cherry Smoothie (recipe in book).

FINAL THOUGHTS ON SPORTS NUTRITION

As a dietitian, my recommendations on sports nutrition are clinical. That means they're based on books, research, and the education I learned in school and through my continuing education. As a licensed, registered medical expert, it's my job to present the "best" evidence-based recommendations for your nutrition.

BUT . . . yes, there's always a but . . . nutrition/health/science is not a one-size-fits-all formula. Each of our bodies are different in so many ways and, in turn, that has an impact on how our body processes food.

This is a long way of saying that everything I say may not work for you when it comes to race nutrition.

Why? Because of what I just said . . . your body is different to my body, which is different to Jeff's body, which is different to the other person reading this book's body. This means that while I can eat an English muffin with peanut butter and run 45 minutes later with no digestive issues, you might not be able to. You may need to wait longer after eating to run. You may need to eat more before you run. Nutrition, especially sports nutrition, is extremely specific to the individual. For that reason, my top tips for sports nutrition are these.

1. You do you. Once you find a sports nutrition strategy that works for you, stick with it. This is a strategy that includes key nutrients, limits gastrointestinal (GI) distress, provides you the energy to complete your activity, and is maintainable long term.

2. Train your sports nutrition. If you have a long run, bike, or race coming up, you train for it. It should not be any different in terms of your sports nutrition. Start practicing the pre-race meal you will have with your longer endurance events. I recommend using a food that you can pack and take with you if you're traveling to a race. You would likely not run a half marathon in new shoes and zero long runs. Why do you take this approach to nutrition and "hope" you figure it out on race day? Your pre-race/run nutrition should be as habitual as charging your watch before a long event. My meal is an English muffin with peanut butter. When I travel for a race, I will pack both so I know my fueling needs are taken care of. Take your pre-run/race nutrition seriously, and this part of your training will see great improvement.

Next, Jeff details his advice on eating and drinking before a long run. His expertise comes not from a nutrition degree but from over 50 years of experience. Both educations are valuable. Learn from what I was taught. Learn from what Jeff knows. Then find a sports nutrition strategy that works for you and stick with it.

PRACTICAL EATING ISSUES—WHAT, WHEN, AND HOW MUCH TO EAT

Jeff Galloway

Carissa covered the nutritional aspects of eating. This section will give you the information and guidelines to deal with the practical issues and problems we have during a workout due to eating. The information is based upon interactions with hundreds of thousands of exercisers to find what works for most.

Most common problems:
1. Eating too much or too soon before workouts.
2. Eating foods that don't digest easily.

Since food eaten up to 4 hours before a workout or race cannot be digested, absorbed, and available for use during the workout, it's best to avoid eating anything before workouts if you have had GI issues during runs.

But if your blood sugar level is low and you want to exercise, a snack can be beneficial. Try various foods to find what works best for you. Simple carbohydrates, even sugar candy, taken within 30 minutes before exercise (about 100 calories) has caused the least problems among my athletes.

If your mouth and or throat are dry, a few sips of water are recommended before short runs. If the exercise lasts less than 90 minutes, it is doubtful that any of the fluid can be absorbed for benefit during the workout. Drinking too much within the 2 hours before a workout can cause more potty stops.

Try out various snacks and strategies of water intake to find what can work for you. But before a 30-to-60-minute workout, you can avoid most problems by not drinking or eating anything.

DURING LONG RUNS, PRACTICE YOUR EATING AND DRINKING STRATEGY

During the 36 hours before a long workout or long event (10K, marathon, half, etc.) the key nutritional goals are 1) to maintain an adequate blood sugar level for daily life activities, and 2) to find foods that don't cause digestive problems when you exercise. Journaling your food intake for a day and a half before long workouts (or speed workouts) can allow you to find the right foods, amounts, and timetable so that you have control over your eating and drinking. Keep fine-tuning so you have a plan for the weekend leading to the big event.

- Thirty-six hours before, eat normal lunch and dinner—if these have not caused problems
- Day before, a normal breakfast and lunch is OK—if you have not had problems with the items before. Try to drink about 8 × 8 ounces of water throughout the day. Avoid salty food
- Afternoon and evening before, taper down on food intake—snack size when hungry
- Evening, avoid a big evening meal and choose foods that have never caused problems when doing long workouts or races
- Avoid alcohol the night before
- Avoid "loading up" with a big meal before a long workout or race as this can lead to "unloading" during the workout or race.

CARBOHYDRATE RELOADING WITHIN 30 MINUTES OF FINISHING

If you don't reload the glycogen with a carbohydrate snack —preferably within 30 minutes of finishing a run—your muscles may not have as much bounce or capacity on the next workout. Those who reload within 30 minutes of finishing a run also report feeling less hungry during the rest of the day. Reload most effectively by eating a snack that has 80 percent carb/20 percent protein based upon the length of your workout or race:

- 100 calories if the race/workout is 4 miles or less
- 300 calories if the race/workout is 13 miles or more
- 100 to 300 calories for in between distances.

NOTE: Use common sense during your evening meal with smaller portions of food that digest easily. Within 15 hours before a strenuous workout, avoid food that tends to cause problems, such as high-fiber foods, fatty or fried foods, and any food that has caused problems for you in the past.

Drinking too much? If you have to take potty stops during walks or runs, you are drinking too much—either before or during the exercise. During an exercise session of 60 minutes or less, most exercisers don't need to drink at all. The intake of fluid before exercise should be arranged so that the excess fluid is eliminated before the run. Each person is a bit different, so you will have to find a routine that works for you.

EATING AND DRINKING TIMETABLE IN THE MORNING OF LONG WORKOUTS OR RACES

- Drink 6 to 8 ounces of water or coffee (180 to 240 milliliters) as soon as you wake up that morning—and that's it until you start the workout.
- If you like to eat something, follow the timetable, and eat items that have not caused problems. (Many exercisers find that they don't need to eat anything before.)
- If you experience low blood sugar as the race/workout start approaches, eat a sugar snack of 100 calories within 30 minutes before the start.
- Reload within 30 minutes after finishing the run: 100 calories for 4 miles or less/300 calories for 13 miles or more.

STOMACH ISSUES DURING LONG RUNS/RACES

Those who have upset stomachs or many toilet stops during long workouts/races should watch the quantity of food eaten the afternoon and evening (day before) and morning of the workout. Practice eating the day before each long run, and journal what, how much, and when. Fine-tune this through the training season and use the successful plan the day before and the morning of your race. Limit fat, high-fiber foods, and avoid eating large portions of meat, poultry, or fish.

DURING WORKOUTS OR RACES

- WATER: 2 to 4 ounces (60–120 milliliters) every 2 miles. Among my athletes, there has been a high percentage of nausea issues when drinking electrolyte beverages during workouts or races.
- BLOOD SUGAR BOOSTING: 30 to 40 calories every 2 miles. Use various snacks during long runs to find the one that works best for you: gummi bears, hard candy, gels, energy bars, sugar cubes have produced the least number of stomach issues among my athletes. (NOTE: Many experienced endurance athletes use de-fizzed soft drinks during long races and workouts—and I do also. One to two sips (2 to 4 ounces) every 2 miles is the guideline.)

PRACTICAL EATING ISSUES

- Diabetics and those with severe hypoglycemia may need to eat more often during long workouts or races. If you need individual help in this area, talk to a registered dietitian.

- Based upon hundreds of reports from runners, I've found that side pain can be caused by ingesting too much fluid or food before exercising.
- If you are running low on blood sugar at the end of your long runs, increase your blood sugar booster snacks from the beginning of your next run.

Long Run/Long Race Eating Schedule

- As soon as you awaken, drink either a cup of coffee or a 6-to-8-ounce glass of water (180 to 240 milliliters).
- Thirty minutes or less before any run (if blood sugar is low), consume approximately 100 calories of a blood sugar booster snack. (If blood sugar is OK, there is no need to consume this snack.)
- Within 30 minutes after a run, consume approximately 100 to 300 calories of an 80 percent carbohydrate/20 percent protein snack.

Hint: Caffeine, when consumed before exercise, engages the systems that enhance running and extend endurance.

EATING AND DRINKING BEFORE AN EVENING EVENT

To ensure the best experience when running at night, you need to focus on what to eat before running at night, and practice it. With proper scheduling of your snacks, you can maintain a good blood sugar level while avoiding nausea from eating too much.

An eating plan: gain control over your energy level and your digestive issues by developing and testing an eating plan during the 5 hours before the race. Here are my suggestions based on the eating success of many runners under similar situations:

- Morning: eat somewhat normally but avoid eating too much. A light breakfast of cereal, or toast with an egg or two egg whites.
- Afternoon: light snacks of 150 to 250 calories, about every 2 hours, with 4 to 6 ounces of water. NOTE: The standard recommendation before various exercise modes is 2 calories per pound of body weight. This seems to work well for cyclists and swimmers, but my runners find that this is a bit too much. Journal your eating before workouts and set up a plan that works for YOU.
- Most find it best to stop eating 2 hours before the run—and many stop eating for a longer period before. Adjust to your needs. If your blood sugar starts to drop, have a light snack, such as an energy bar, gummi bears (no more than 150 calories, 30 minutes before the race).

- Avoid snacks that are high in fat or high in fiber. Choose foods that are easy to digest.
- Drink 4 to 6 ounces (120 to 180 milliliters) of water with each snack (or coffee if you like it).
- Blood sugar insurance. Carry a bag of blood sugar booster snacks, such as gummi bears, hard candies, sugar cubes, or the sugar source of your choice to consume during the half hour before the start—in case your blood sugar level drops.
- Blood sugar snacks during the long runs/races. My rule of thumb is 30 to 40 calories every 2 miles. Try this and fine-tune to your needs. Bring a bag of the snacks that you have used successfully, and you can maintain control over low blood sugar.

Fluids:

- Morning: 6 to 8 ounces (180 to 240 milliliters) of water every hour. One 8-ounce drink could be an electrolyte beverage.
- Afternoon: Drink 4 to 6 ounces (120 to 180 milliliters) of water or electrolyte beverage every hour—or with each snack.
- During the 2 hours before long runs or the race, it's best to stop drinking or minimize fluid intake (so that you can take your potty stop before the start of the run, instead of during the run).
- Avoid alcohol before the race.
- Caffeine is generally OK if you are used to consuming it before runs. Generally it's best to drink your last caffeinated beverage about 2 hours before the start, but do what works for you.
- The rule of thumb during the race is 2 to 4 ounces of water, every 2 miles. Don't drink more than 20 ounces an hour.
- Enjoy every mile and the party afterward.

PRACTICE RUNNING AND EATING IN THE EVENING

Practice by running in the evening two to three times. During the training period, schedule at least two of your runs at about the time the race will start. This will help you adjust to running at night. Journal what you eat before the start, and edit according to the results.

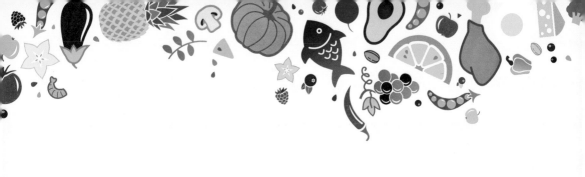

CHAPTER 4

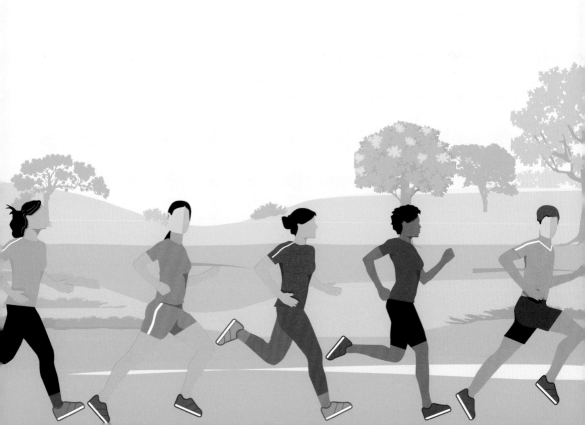

NUTRITION MYTHS AND FAQS

Nutrition information is everywhere! Books, TV, social media, your neighbor . . . It's time to separate the fact from the fiction and explain how these myths really impact you!

Carissa Galloway, RDN

MARATHON TRAINING AND WEIGHT GAIN

MYTH: MARATHON TRAINING CAN CAUSE YOU TO GAIN WEIGHT

True or false? TRUE, but that's OK!

While many people start marathon training with a goal of weight loss, it often doesn't work out that way. True. Marathon training can cause weight gain, but it doesn't have to.

I'm sure you've heard stories about many people who take up running or walking and lose weight. If you are one of these people, then congrats! You are getting the physical and mental benefits of exercise, and keep doing what you're doing!

When you go from limited physical activity to regular exercise of over 30 minutes, or more, your body makes many positive adaptations. One of which is an increased caloric expenditure. If, with that extra activity, your daily caloric intake remains, then you will likely lose weight.

The longer you exercise and the more often you run, means your body has different needs and might make slightly different adaptations.

If you have trained for a marathon properly, you know this is a big, courageous endeavor. Even with the most moderate plans, you are running at least 3 days a week with long runs that can take 5 hours depending on your pace. Training for a marathon is a big deal, and it's a big deal to your body as well. Simple math would say that if you run for 5 hours you'll burn thousands of calories and you should lose weight . . . however, reality says that isn't always the case and physiologically there are a few reasons why.

- We can easily "out eat" a long run
  - » It's easy to overestimate the number of calories you burn during a long run and then overeat after that long run. The average person will burn between 80 and 140 calories per mile. Most of the tracking devices we use will overestimate how many calories we burn. If your 10-mile training run burns 1,000 calories, and you had 200 calories of nutrition during the run, and you have a big breakfast afterwards, then you have essentially used up the calorie deficit you created during the run. And that's ok! You need to refuel, but be aware that a fancy latte, four pancakes, three eggs, and a side of fruit is likely over 1,000 calories.
- Constantly rewarding yourself with food
  - » "I ran so far . . . I can have another slice of pizza." The longer we run, the more we open the reward circuits of our brain. I get it—that run was hard and you want to be rewarded! Don't make food your reward. Reward yourself for your hard work with a pedicure, spa time, new workout clothes, or by booking a destination race. This will keep your focus on the benefits of the runs and not food as a reward.
- Extra calories needed for training
  - » When you have runs lasting over an hour you will need to increase your caloric intake. As discussed in chapter 3, you need to add in extra carbohydrates in the days leading up to a long run to prime your glycogen stores. This makes sure you have the energy to complete your run. You also need to take in calories during your run to sustain your energy.
  - » These calories are needed. If weight loss is your goal, please don't eliminate these calories as it will negatively impact your ability to perform and train and increase your risk of injury.
- You're eating more carbs
  - » You're eating more carbohydrates to fuel yourself to train for a marathon. That's smart! However, your body needs to store those carbs as glycogen. Your body typically stores this glycogen in your liver, and this causes your body to hold onto more water to make that glycogen available to you. For every ounce of glycogen stored, your body also stores about 3 ounces of water. This leads to extra water weight, which you will notice on the scale. Don't panic, don't cut carbs. Your body needs these to run and help you reach your goal.
- Early run disrupting regular sleep
  - » Many runners use the early morning hours to get in training runs. This may decrease the amount of sleep you get regularly and make you tired. When you're tired research has shown you're more likely to mindlessly eat and

crave carbohydrates. Your body, when tired, releases the stress hormone cortisol, which also causes the body to hold onto weight.

» Make slight adjustments to your sleep schedule to accommodate training. Turn off electronics one hour before bed and, if you can, take a post-long-run nap. Talk about a well-deserved reward that's not food!

- Physiological adaptations to training

» As marathon training continues, your body will gain strength, which means you gain muscle. Again, this is a good thing as your body prepares for your 26.2-mile race. While muscle does not weigh more than fat (1 pound of muscle = 1 pound of fat), it is a denser tissue. As you gain muscle, the scale may go up; however, since muscle is denser than fat, you may notice a leaner overall appearance, which most athletes see as a positive change!

Based on all the above, I recommend that if you are strictly trying to lose weight, stick to a lighter running schedule. When you're ready to tackle a marathon, let that be the focus and use the nutrition knowledge you've gained here to keep your food choices education based.

If you are thinking about training for a half marathon or marathon and you want to lose weight, please DO NOT let this deter you. It is possible, and now you are armed with the scientific information to make choices that allow your body to adapt to the training it needs to complete a marathon and make smart nutrition choices.

MYTH: I CAN SKIP BREAKFAST BEFORE A LONG RUN

FALSE!

I hope that after reading the first few chapters of this book, I have convinced you of the many benefits of carbohydrates in your diet. If you are doing a run over 45 to 60 minutes, then not only do you need to fuel your body with carbohydrates before the run but you must plan to rehydrate and consume simple, easily digested carbohydrates while you're exercising. Without doing this, you risk injury, decreased performance, and mental struggles due to lack of energy. It will be harder for you to accomplish your long run if you don't fuel!

There are some of you reading this who are shaking your head, saying that you can't eat before you run. The stomach is a finicky organ, and I do understand; however, I must implore you to train your nutrition before a long run, just like you

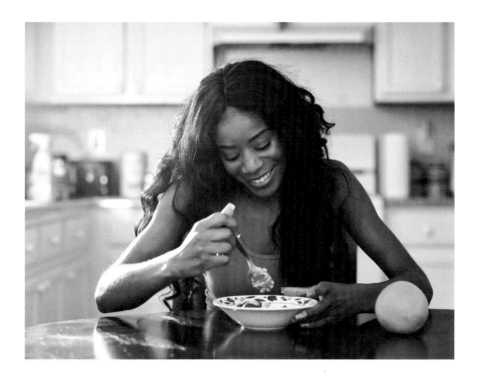

train to run a race. Try eating earlier before you run, or try eating something easier to digest like crackers or a sports gel closer to when you run. Practice your nutrition, and, over time, you will find a strategy that works for you and lets you get in the necessary calories for activity. I suggest using a notebook to record what and when you eat before a long run. Make notes on how the activity goes and use this to make adjustments to your pre-run meal until you're able to tolerate at least 200 to 300 calories, 1 to 2 hours before the run, with the goal being 200 to 300 grams of carbohydrates 3 to 4 hours before a long activity.

If you don't tolerate food well before a run try:

- 4 to 6 ounces of sports drink 30 minutes before you run
- ½ cup of dry cereal
- Banana
- Dried fruit, such as dates or raisins
- Typical in-run fuel like GUs, chews, etc.

MYTH: I CAN SKIP BREAKFAST BEFORE A SHORT (LESS THAN 45 MINUTE) WORKOUT

Sometimes TRUE!

Shorter, lower-intensity exercise is possible on an empty stomach. Some nutrition experts may argue otherwise, but I won't tell you to do anything I don't do myself. When I am doing an easy workout in the morning that's less than 30 minutes, I will often have coffee and nothing else. This is usually because I am not a morning person, and I don't have time to eat and wait to digest.

When you are in a fasted state, your body will primarily use fat for energy, which can be a benefit for weight loss. My recommendation when fasting before cardio is to keep it under 45 minutes and keep the intensity low. Don't go over a level where you cannot easily carry on a conversation.

If you have a tough workout like hill repeats or intervals, then I recommend a small snack like fruit, dry cereal, or toast. The carbohydrates will give you more energy, which will improve your effort during the workout. This will lead to benefits in your training.

MYTH: I WILL LOSE WEIGHT ON A LOW-CARB DIET

TRUE . . . but . . .

Yes, when you cut out carbohydrates from your diet you will lose weight. Likely this initial weight loss is water weight. Remember those 3 ounces of water that your body stores with glycogen? When you limit carbohydrates, your body reaches into its glycogen stores for energy, and as this glycogen is used the water is released, you will see a decrease in your weight on the scale. However, if you are training for a long race or looking to improve your athletic performance, you need these glycogen stores, and a dramatically reduced carbohydrate diet might make training more challenging.

As a dietitian, I do not recommend diets that cut or severely limit one food group. I find that low-carb diets are a challenging diet to stay on long term. This is especially true for active people whose bodies will crave the quick energy boost that carbs bring. Carbs are not bad. Carbs alone do not cause weight gain. Carbs can have many beneficial nutrients like B-vitamins, potassium, fiber, and folate. It's okay to eat carbs!

MYTH: A VEGETARIAN DIET WON'T MEET MY NUTRIENT NEEDS

FALSE.

A well-balanced vegetarian diet can meet not only your nutrient needs but research says it may be beneficial to your overall health and longevity and can reduce your risk of heart disease, diabetes, and some cancers.

There are five main variations of vegetarian diets:

- **Lacto-vegetarian** diets exclude meat, fish, poultry, and eggs, as well as foods that contain them. Dairy products, such as milk, cheese, yogurt, and butter, are included.
- **Ovo-vegetarian** diets exclude meat, poultry, seafood, and dairy products, but allow eggs.
- **Lacto-ovo vegetarian** diets exclude meat, fish, and poultry, but allow dairy products and eggs.
- **Pescatarian** diets exclude meat and poultry, dairy, and eggs, but allow fish.
- **Vegan** diets exclude meat, poultry, fish, eggs, and dairy products, and foods that contain these products.

If you choose a vegetarian diet, make sure to aim for variety and build the base of your diet on fruits, vegetables, beans, whole grain carbohydrates, and calcium-rich foods. Some vegetarian diets can rely too much on heavily processed, carbohydrate-rich foods.

Here are five nutrients to focus on if you follow a vegetarian diet:

1. Calcium
    - Calcium is easily found in dairy foods. Calcium can also be found in plant sources although these are not as well absorbed by the body.
    - Sources of calcium include:
        » Low-fat or fat-free milk, yogurt, and cheese
        » Fortified plant-based milks, such as soy or almond
        » Fortified cereals
        » Calcium-fortified juice
        » Some leafy green vegetables including collard greens, turnip greens, and kale
        » Broccoli
        » Beans including soybeans, chickpeas, and black beans
        » Almonds and almond butter.

2. Iron
   - Aim to consume a variety of iron-rich foods each day and pair it with a source of vitamin C to boost absorption.
   - Sources of iron include:
     » Legumes such as beans, peas, and lentils
     » Eggs
     » Whole grains
     » Soy products
     » Nuts and nut butters
     » Some dairy products.
3. Protein
   - Most vegetarians who consume a well-balanced diet and plenty of protein throughout the day will have an adequate protein intake.
   - Vegetarian sources of protein include:
     » Beans, peas, and lentils
     » Whole grains
     » Meat alternatives like Beyond or Impossible Foods
     » Soy products
     » Nuts and nut butters
     » Dairy products
     » Eggs.
4. Vitamin B12
   - B12 is a more challenging nutrient to find in a vegetarian diet as it is commonly found in animal products. I recommend that all vegetarians, and especially vegans, choose foods fortified with vitamin B12 and ask their medical provider if a vitamin B12 (cobalamin) supplement is needed.
   - Vegetarian sources of B12 include:
     » Nutritional yeast
     » Soy milk
     » Meat substitutes
     » Ready-to-eat cereals (check the label)
     » Eggs.
5. Vitamin D
   - Vitamin D is found in very few foods. It's mainly found in dairy foods. If you are a vegan or do not get adequate sunlight, then also check with your medical provider about the need for a vitamin D supplement.
   - Vegetarian sources of vitamin D include:
     » Eggs
     » Vitamin D fortified foods including milk, orange juice, cereals, and soy milk
     » Mushrooms that have been exposed to UV light.

As I mentioned in the protein section at the start of the book, most Americans get plenty of protein, and protein recommendations are lower than most of us think.

COMMONLY ASKED NUTRITION QUESTIONS

DO YOU RECOMMEND INTERMITTENT FASTING?

Over the past few years, this has become one of the questions I am asked the most. My answer depends on several factors:

* What length of fasting?
* What are your fitness goals? Are you training for a longer event?
* Are you in menopause?

Those answers will determine if I think you could possibly benefit from intermittent fasting.

My second point is always to emphasize that if you take part in intermittent fasting, that does not mean that you can eat junk during your eating window. You still need to consume a diet balanced with fruits, vegetables, fiber, whole grains, and lean protein.

I'M GETTING OLDER AND WORRIED ABOUT MY BONE HEALTH.
WHAT IS ONE VITAMIN THAT YOU CAN TAKE FOR STRONGER BONES?

Calcium is a main factor in bone development, and a diet low in calcium during a person's lifetime can increase their risk for osteoporosis. Vitamin D is equally important due to its effect on calcium. If your body is lacking in vitamin D, you are unable to absorb the calcium you consume from foods. Aim to include both calcium and vitamin D daily in your diet and aim to have sources in multiple meals. Foods that are high in calcium include dairy products, green, leafy vegetables, tofu, almonds, salmon, and sardines (eat the bones!). Many foods are fortified with vitamin D and calcium, and these are highly recommended and can include things like orange juice, cereals, bread, and protein shakes.

Dietary proteins also contain nutrients needed for bone health and, as such, can help prevent osteoporosis. Maintaining a diet that is adequate in protein will support bone health. Choose protein sources that also have calcium such as dairy, tofu, salmon, and protein powders. It's also worth noting that exercise, specifically weight-bearing exercise, is critical to building and maintaining strong bones.

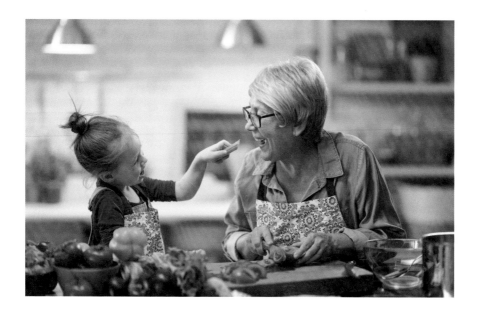

DO YOU RECOMMEND PROTEIN SHAKES AFTER A WORKOUT? WHEN SHOULD I DRINK THEM, AND WHAT TYPE OF PROTEIN?

To see the best results from the effort you put into your workouts you should refuel with protein and carbohydrates. Whole-food protein sources and protein powders and drinks will both serve the same purpose of providing your body with the amino acids it needs. You will see the most benefits to recovery and muscle synthesis by consuming a high-quality protein within 90 minutes of your workout.

WHAT'S THE BEST PROTEIN POWDER POST WORKOUT?

If your goal is recovery and rebuilding after a workout, look for a protein that is whey-based. Whey protein is one of the best post-workout protein options. Why? Whey protein sends amino acids to muscles quickly to jump-start muscle growth. There is also research that supports combining whey and casein powders post workout as this duo can speed not only the uptake of amino acids but also extend their absorption.

It's important to remember that you can consume too much protein at one time, which means it will be less effective. Your body can effectively absorb 25 to 35 grams of protein in one sitting, so aim for your serving to be no more than 35 grams of protein.

I FIND I OFTEN HAVE TROUBLE SLEEPING ESPECIALLY BEFORE A LONG RUN OR RACE. ARE THERE ANY FOODS THAT CAN HELP ME SLEEP BETTER?

Almonds—When we think of a natural way to support sleep, many of us think of melatonin. Almonds are one type of nut that contains melatonin. If you're hungry before bed, a handful of almonds is a low-carb way to boost satiety and increase melatonin, which helps signal your body to prepare for sleep.

Tart Cherry Juice—As an athlete, I was drawn to learning more about tart cherry juice as it relates to recovery and inflammation, but another benefit of frequent consumption that has been proven by science is sleep benefit. Not only does tart cherry juice boost your body's production of melatonin but it also increases the bioavailability of tryptophan. Tryptophan is then used to make serotonin, which calms us down and helps us sleep.

Chamomile Tea—There are numerous studies to support ways that chamomile tea can support a healthy nighttime routine. Aside from other health benefits of chamomile tea, it contains the antioxidant apigenin. Apigenin connects with receptors in our brains to reduce insomnia and promote a state of steady sleep. Try chamomile tea 1 hour before bed, and give it up to 2 weeks to notice positive changes.

Banana With Peanut Butter—Foods with unsaturated fats like peanut butter will improve serotonin levels and help boost satiety to keep you feeling satisfied and not hungry during sleep. Bananas can be a good vehicle for peanut butter before bed as they contain magnesium, which can also support good sleep. Magnesium plays a role in sleep regulation and can also help support a sense of relaxation and calm.

I'M ALWAYS BEING SERVED ADS ABOUT "DRINK MIX-INS LIKE COLLAGEN OR LIQUID GREENS." DO THESE ACTUALLY WORK?

Like any food, drink, or wellness mix-in, it totally depends on what the product is. There are plenty of legitimate mix-ins out there that will support your overall health, but there are also some built on hype that won't do much apart from give you an expensive drink. Before you buy a mix-in, do your research. Check out any research about the supplement and read reviews from those who have purchased it. Also look at how many calories or how many grams of sodium and fat the mix-in might add. We tend to not scrutinize mix-ins as much as we would other foods, so make sure what you're adding in fits into your dietary goals.

As a runner, I'm a fan of electrolyte mix-ins. They offer a convenient way to replenish electrolytes lost after exercise, which is essential. I also like adding collagen to my hot tea or morning smoothie. Collagen has a range of benefits, from skin health to bone and joint health. There have been some concerns raised about possibly denaturing collagen by adding it to a hot beverage; however, as long as the drink is above 300°F, it should not damage the protein.

One type of mix-in that I tend not to recommend are those designed to give you a daily intake of "greens" or vegetables. Most fresh produce, fruits and vegetables both, will give you the maximum nutrition when eaten as a whole food. In a powdered source not only do you not get the highly valuable fiber from the plant, but many of the vitamins and minerals could be less effective when taken in a powdered form.

I LOVE DRINKING SWEETENED COFFEE AND I KNOW COFFEE HAS SOME HEALTH BENEFITS. IS THERE A WAY TO ENJOY COFFEE WITHOUT THE EXCESS CALORIES THAT ADD FLAVOR?

Most dietitians will tell you that a daily 300-calorie latte might not be the best habit if you're looking to lose weight or reach other wellness goals. BUT that doesn't mean that all coffee drinks are off-limits. Coffee on its own, as we know, is very low calorie, about 1 calorie per cup of black coffee. Therefore, the issue isn't the coffee, but what you put in it.

An update to try is Proffee. Proffee = protein + coffee. Next time you visit the coffee house skip the seasonal high-sugar latte and ask for two shots of espresso on ice in a venti cup. Then add a ready-to-drink protein shake (my favorite is a caramel shake) to the ice and espresso. Now you have your coffee with satisfying protein instead of sugar, which would spike your blood sugar. The Proffee trend is perfect for after your morning workout, and it's also a favorite of healthcare workers who work long hours without time to stop for full meals; Proffee gives them energy to power through their day fueled by java and protein.

CHAPTER 5

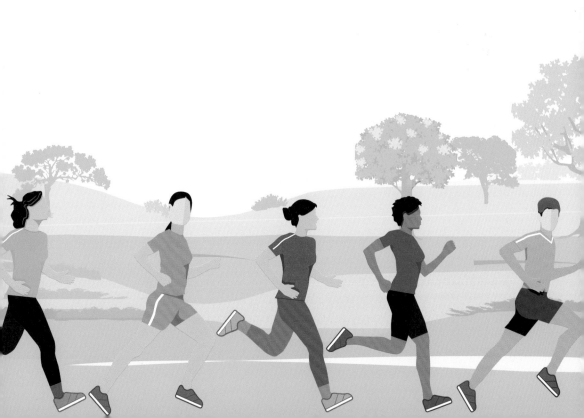

FOODS YOU'RE NOT EATING ENOUGH OF AND WHY

Simple swaps can make a big impact on your diet—add these foods into your diet NOW!

Carissa Galloway, RDN

It can seem overwhelming to feel that you have to change your entire diet to improve your health. You don't! You can make simple swaps or "upgrades," as I like to call them, to your current diet, and those changes over time really can make a big difference. This chapter will cover all my recommended foods to include in your diet and easy ways to swap them for foods you might already be eating.

FOODS YOU SHOULD EAT MORE OFTEN

CHIA SEEDS

There are several reasons why chia seeds are healthy, but the main one is linked to the 11 grams of fiber they offer in a 1-ounce serving. When we increase the fiber in our diet, it can help regulate blood cholesterol levels and naturally lower blood pressure. Chia seeds are also a vegetarian source of omega-3 fatty acids, which can help reduce total body inflammation, reduce stress throughout the body, and thus prevent strain on blood vessels, which aids in the prevention of heart disease. It is worth noting that you still need to add omega-3s with docosahexaenoic acid (DHA) into your diet as chia seeds supply omega-3s with alpha-linolenic acid (AHA), and not DHA. Chia seeds also contain antioxidants and are a vegetarian source of high-quality protein.

Unlike flax seeds, chia seeds can be eaten raw to receive all their benefits. You can add them raw into smoothies, salads, or in a muffin mix. In vegan baking, they are used to replace eggs, and my mother-in-law makes them into a gel to keep her turkey burgers moist.

FLAXSEEDS

Flaxseeds have a reputation as one of the healthiest foods on the planet, and there's evidence of them being consumed as early as 3000 BC. Research shows that the plant omega-3s in flaxseeds can support heart health through anti-inflammatory actions and normalizing heart rate, similar to chia seeds. New research also shows support for flaxseeds to aid in naturally lowering blood pressure. Also, as with chia seeds and oatmeal, the fiber in flaxseeds is beneficial for lowering LDL cholesterol. Specifically, in flaxseeds the cholesterol-lowering benefits can be attributed to the trio of omega-3 ALA, lignans, and fiber.

To make the most of your flaxseed consumption, don't eat it whole. If eaten before being ground, the flaxseed is more likely to pass through your intestinal tract undigested and your body will not absorb all its health benefits. In terms of a name, milled flaxseed, ground flaxseed, and flax meal all refer to the same thing. Also, when looking at flaxseed added into products, make sure you check the label says it is "ground" flaxseed. It's best to store ground flaxseed in the freezer to maintain its omega-3 properties.

You can use ground flaxseed as an additive to smoothies and baked goods. I use it in my breading for baked chicken parmesan, and I also add 2 tablespoons to my black bean chili. Nobody notices, and the health benefits just add up!

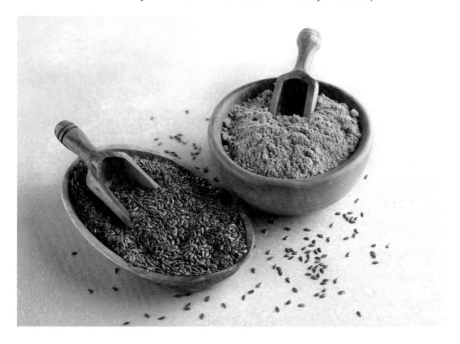

LENTILS

Lentils aren't as popular as beans, but they're just as much of a health food superstar. You don't need to soak them before you cook them. Substitute them for meat in soups or stews, and you'll get a hearty boost of protein and fiber for a lot less fat. They are also a very affordable protein source.

PRUNES/DRIED PLUMS

Prunes, which are dried plums, do much more than keep your digestion regular. They're also high in antioxidants and fiber. Recent research shows that eating five or six prunes a day can support bone health. For prunes, a quarter-cup has 104 calories and 12 percent of the fiber you need in a day. You can eat them as-is, chop them up and add them to muffins or other baked goods, or include them in smoothies, cereals, sauces, or stews. I like to use these when I travel as a snack and to help digestion.

ARTICHOKES

Have you tried artichokes? They rank highest among antioxidants in vegetables. You can grill them, bake them, and eat the leaves or the heart. Finish off the whole artichoke and you'll only get about 60 calories and almost no fat, not counting any dip or sauce you ate it with. High in fiber, it will fill you up so you won't splurge on higher-fat foods. Time to think past the spinach artichoke dip! For an easy way to cook artichokes at home, use an instant pot.

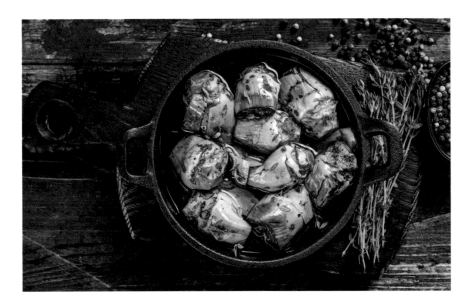

BEETS

Be one with the beet! These brightly colored root vegetables look rough on the outside, but they're softer and sweeter once you cook them. Beets are high in antioxidants, which may help protect against cancer and other chronic diseases. Plus their juice, which is rich in nitrates, has been found to lower blood pressure and increase blood flow to the brain. If you're an athlete, snacking on beets might even help improve your performance.

SEAWEED

Unless you're a fan of sushi, seaweed may never have passed your lips. But this member of the algae family is definitely worth a try. Because it absorbs nutrients from the sea, seaweed is rich in many vitamins and minerals, especially calcium and iron. It's also high in protein and low in fat. Try seaweed snacks as an alternative to potato chips.

CAULIFLOWER

Broccoli is the relative that gets all the attention, but its paler cousin is no wallflower. Like other cruciferous veggies, cauliflower is a good source of vitamin C and fiber. Like broccoli, it also has a natural plant chemical called sulforaphane that may hold promise against cancer, according to early lab tests in animals. Many other things also affect your cancer risk, but diet is one of the easiest to control.

PROBIOTICS

Treat your gut well! Gut health and immune health are interconnected. Probiotics can help support a healthy digestive tract so consider taking a daily probiotic or eating foods high in probiotics like yogurt with live, active cultures, or fermented foods. *Lactobacillus* strains to look for that support digestive and immune health include *L. brevis, L. casei, L. paracasei,* and *L. salivarius.*

Good sources of probiotics to include in your diet daily include yogurt with live and active cultures (note: read the label, it needs to say this for it to have beneficial probiotics), kombucha and kefir. Probiotics are live, so they won't live in your digestive tract doing their beneficial work endlessly. Aim to consume one of these sources of probiotics daily or supplement with a probiotic capsule.

Kombucha is another way to get living probiotics into your diet, and I like to drink a kombucha as an afternoon pick me up. You can also get probiotics from yogurt. Make sure to check on the label that the yogurt contains live, active cultures.

KEFIR

This bubbly form of fermented milk has been a dietary staple in the Caucasus Mountains of Eastern Europe for many years. Recently, it's started to catch on in the United States that kefir is high in "good" bacteria, aka probiotics. It is also being studied for its anti-inflammatory and anti-cancer effects.

FOODS FOR IMMUNITY

For the past few years, immunity is a word we've heard repeatedly. We want to boost our immunity against any invader/virus/bacteria/stressor that can cause our bodies harm. What we eat has a major impact on our immunity.

I could make this list very short and tell you that eating more fruits and vegetables will support your immune system. It's true. Simply eating more fruits and vegetables will boost your immunity, and also make it easier to maintain a healthy weight, prevent certain cancers, lower your bad cholesterol . . . Plants do a lot. Eat more.

If immunity is top of mind, then add these foods to your grocery list and consume regularly. Remember, an orange you eat March 1 will do little to support your immunity in the middle of May. To get the benefits of these foods, make sure to regularly consume them or regularly consume foods that contain similar micronutrients.

CITRUS FRUITS

As we think about immunity, vitamin C is a micronutrient that will be talked about a lot. Vitamin C is a water-soluble vitamin, which among other things, plays a role in supporting a healthy immune system. Vitamin C is an essential vitamin meaning your body can't make it, so you must get it from food to get all the impressive benefits. Vitamin C is an antioxidant that keeps your immune system strong by protecting your body from free radicals. Vitamin C also supports the production of white blood cells called lymphocytes and phagocytes. These are cells that work to protect your body against infection. Research has shown that low vitamin C levels are indicative of poorer health outcomes.

Citrus fruits are easy ways to get vitamin C because they're portable, affordable, and can be consumed daily. Pick whole fruits over juices to get the benefits of the fiber in the whole fruits.

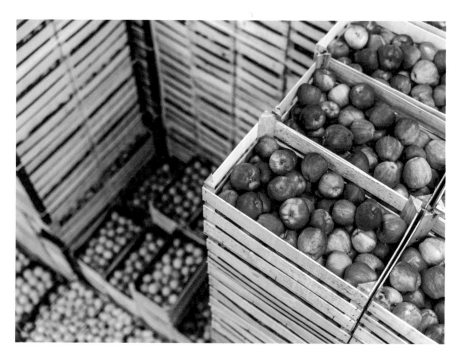

I like easy-to-peel mandarins as a snack, but you can also add citrus into a spinach salad or use the juice in a marinade with other immune-boosting foods, such as garlic and ginger.

APPLES

Apple skin contains quercetin, which is a phytochemical that can support immune health and reduce inflammation. Don't forget to eat the peel for these benefits. Additionally, apples have pectin, which is a prebiotic and promotes gut health. As we learn more about our gut, we see the connection between a healthy gut and immunity. I make gut health a part of my wellness goals all year long by making sure I'm getting both pre- and probiotics. Apples have vitamin C, and all the benefits of citrus fruits apply to apples, however, citrus fruits tend to have a higher percentage of vitamin C than apples.

Apples are a great portable snack. I regularly tell all my clients (and anyone who will listen) to eat an apple a day on an empty stomach. Think of an apple as a "toothbrush" for your inside. The fiber will help your digestion and your cholesterol. For another easy way to enjoy apples, I like to add diced apples to oatmeal and top with cinnamon for an "apple pie" breakfast combination. You can also add diced apples to a Waldorf-inspired salad using rotisserie chicken for a make ahead lunch.

PEARS

Pears contain vitamin C, which helps support a healthy immune system. Immune support is just one of the benefits that vitamin C has been linked to. Other benefits include helping to lower blood pressure and levels of the stress hormone cortisol. Pears also have phytochemical compounds in their peels like apples, which support immune health by fighting free radicals. Pears contain a significant amount of vitamin A and, along with vitamin C, this can help our body stimulate the production of white blood cells, which strengthens the immune system. Pears have fiber and prebiotics like apples, which supports healthy digestion and boosts gut health.

Pears are great in many of the ways apples are. They are great in a salad, sprinkled with cinnamon for a sweet treat, or on a snack platter with an ounce of sliced cheddar cheese.

CRANBERRIES

Cranberry juice is rich in vitamin C, which supports the immune system and helps it continue to function normally. Cranberry juice can be high in sugar so check the nutrition label and avoid buying cranberry juice "cocktail" as it likely won't have the 100 percent cranberry juice needed for these benefits.

The skin of cranberries contains many powerful antioxidants like quercetin; however, cranberry juice doesn't contain high amounts of cranberry skin, so aim for dried or even fresh cranberries to maximize the immune benefits. Cranberries contain polyphenols and bioactive plant compounds that research has linked with a reduction of inflammation, among other benefits like improved heart and digestive health.

SALMON

Getting enough healthy fats in your diet can bolster your own body's immune response by decreasing overall inflammation. Low-level inflammation is common and is a typical response to injury or stress; however, the concern is chronic inflammation, which can have a negative, suppressing effect on your immune system. Healthy fats like olive oil and omega-3 fatty acids are anti-inflammatory; thus, the connection can be made that they will naturally fight illness with their anti-inflammatory properties. Salmon is high in omega-3s, so adding omega-3-rich seafood into your diet at least twice a week can support immune health. For a simple salmon dish, I top salmon filets with olive oil (another immune-boosting and anti-inflammatory fat) with salt, pepper, herbs, and fresh lemon juice. Bake salmon in a 400°F oven for 20 to 25 minutes until cooked to your desired level of doneness.

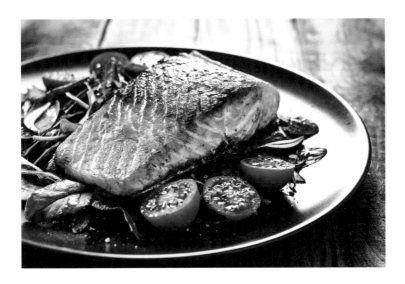

FOODS THAT IMPROVE MOOD

Let food be thy medicine. Just as a high-fat meal can make us feel sluggish and not at our best, there are other foods that support or boost our mood biologically. All these are foods are praised in this book. This is just another nudge to include them in your diet frequently.

SALMON

High concentrations of omega-3 fatty acids—the heart-healthy fats that aid mood and memory—are present in the brain. Salmon is chock-full of omega-3s, and University of Maryland Medical Center researchers suggest that these nutrients can help lift mood, alleviate mild depression, and improve memory as well. I love salmon as an easy weeknight dinner and roast it in the oven alongside asparagus for a one-pan meal and a mood boost!

EGGS

An egg contains countless nutrients to help support a healthy body and mind. Although egg yolks are commonly shunned for their high cholesterol content, they're also rich in good-for-you nutrients like vitamins D, B12, and choline; nutrients that are all important for brain development and function. Additionally, eggs have selenium, and a selenium deficiency has been linked to depression and poor mood.

LEAFY GREENS

Dark leafy greens—such as spinach, turnip greens and romaine lettuce—are high in folic acid, a nutrient that the National Institutes of Health report as alleviating depression and reducing fatigue. (The asparagus I mentioned before alongside the salmon is also high in folic acid so another great choice for mood food.)

MILK

The Mayo Clinic suggests that consuming whey, a protein present in milk, may decrease anxiety and stress. You can find whey protein in many protein powders and yogurt, ricotta and cottage cheese.

WHOLE GRAINS

Carbohydrates tend to top the list of comfort foods for a lot of people, and there's science behind the reason why. One theory surrounding why you crave carbohydrates is low serotonin levels. Carbs are thought to boost the production of these mood-regulating chemicals. Choose carbs rich in fiber—for example, oatmeal, legumes, and whole grains—they can help you maintain your weight and beat the bad mood blues. Start your day with whole-grain toast topped with avocado for another trending way to boost your mood.

CHOCOLATE

The boost in mood you get when you treat yourself is not a coincidence. According to research, chocolate makes you feel good because it's full of a mix of mood-elevating chemicals, including caffeine, theobromine, tyrosine, and tryptophan. For even more benefits, choose dark chocolate and enjoy the antioxidant boost.

BANANAS

I had a chemistry professor who told me that monkeys were happy because they ate bananas, and maybe he wasn't wrong. Bananas contain tryptophan, which is a protein that is converted to mood-boosting serotonin in the body. Bananas aren't only good after a run; I like them topped with nut butter for a midday snack with a few dark chocolate chips.

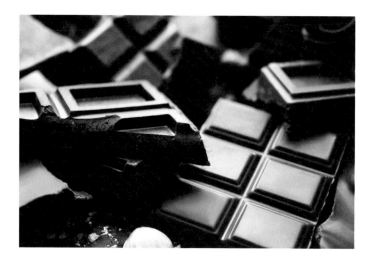

WALNUTS

All nuts do well at helping to balance your blood sugar levels, which can help decrease mood swings. I like walnuts because they have two nutrients that we previously talked about that support mood: magnesium and omega-3 fatty acids.

BERRIES

The bright color of berries is linked with many health benefits and related to the antioxidants contained in them. One specific antioxidant, anthocyanin, has been associated with a decreased risk of depression symptoms, so add dark purple-blue berries to your shopping list to top an oatmeal bowl or spinach and berry salad.

 MORE ON ANTIOXIDANTS

AVOCADO

Avocados also make the list for several of the nutrients we've talked about before. When you reach for an avocado, you're getting omega-3s, folate, and tryptophan. No wonder taco Tuesday makes us all smile!

SPINACH

Spinach is packed with several of the nutrients we've previously discussed that support immunity. Spinach is rich in vitamin C and antioxidants like vitamin A.

Most Americans aren't getting enough vegetables in their daily diet, so feel free to incorporate this beneficial leafy green whenever you can. Add spinach into your morning smoothie, top a lunch sandwich with spinach, and sauté it in heart-healthy olive oil alongside roasted salmon for a satisfying, immune-boosting dinner.

GREEN TEA

A simple way to support your body's immune system is by incorporating green tea into your daily routine. Green tea contains flavonoids, which are a type of antioxidant. Green tea specifically contains high amounts of the antioxidant epigallocatechin gallate (ECGC), which has been shown to enhance immune function. As you enjoy your green tea, be mindful of added sugars, and aim to enjoy the taste without sugar as often as possible. If you're adding green tea into your diet, aim for two sugar-free cups per day.

POTASSIUM-FILLED FOODS TO LOWER BLOOD PRESSURE

Many Americans are plagued by high blood pressure, and the medical community often turns to medication to lower blood pressure. High blood pressure increases your risk of heart attack and stroke among other things, so I am not opposed to medication to prevent that, however, wouldn't it be nice to lower your blood pressure naturally?

Reducing sodium in your diet will make a big impact on lowering blood pressure. Adding in foods with potassium will as well, and I just love how adding nutritious foods into our diets can help heal our bodies. You don't just have to take foods OUT of your diet to improve your health. Add in any of the following potassium-rich foods to support lowering blood pressure naturally. Potassium can also prevent the formation of kidney stones and help maintain bone density. Potassium is an electrolyte too, so these foods help your body recover after exercise too!

Good sources of potassium include:

- Baked sweet potato: 694 milligrams
- Tomato paste (¼ cup): 664 milligrams
- Non-fat plain yogurt (8 ounces): 579 milligrams
- Banana: 487 milligrams
- Yellowfin tuna (3 ounces): 484 milligrams
- Kidney beans (½ cup): 356 milligrams
- Spinach (2 cups raw): 335 milligrams.

CALCIUM

Calcium is the most abundant mineral in your body, and like potassium, it can also help naturally lower blood pressure. Calcium is most known for its connection to bone health, so as we age, especially women, we need to make sure we're getting enough calcium to support bone health. Calcium is also needed to maintain heart rhythm and muscle function, and consuming enough dietary calcium may reduce the risk of obesity.

Calcium needs change as we age. Adults up to age 50 need 1,000 milligrams/ day. That increases as we age. Adults over age 50 need 1,200 milligrams/day. Those with a higher risk of osteoporosis may need up to 1,500 milligrams/day. For reference, one serving of dairy will contain about 300 milligrams of calcium.

Good sources of calcium include:

- Non-fat plain yogurt (8 ounces): 452 milligrams
- Swiss cheese (1.5 ounces): 336 milligrams
- Skim milk (8 ounces): 306 milligrams
- Salmon (3 ounces): 181 milligrams
- Cooked spinach (1 cup): 146 milligrams
- Calcium is also in all sorts of fortified foods, such as breakfast cereals, orange juice, and soy milk.

MAGNESIUM

Are you looking for more ways to lower blood pressure naturally? Then think about magnesium. Many of us don't think about magnesium in our diets often, but it has many benefits. Personally, I take a magnesium supplement when traveling to support my healthy digestion and mood. Magnesium is also needed for proper metabolism, to strengthen bones, boost immunity, and maintain a regular heartbeat. There's also research to support a link between magnesium intake and a reduced risk of Type 2 diabetes. Choosing heart-healthy nuts is a great way to boost the magnesium intake in your diet as are the following options.

- Brazil nuts (1 ounce): 107 milligrams
- 100 percent bran cereal (1 ounce): 103 milligrams
- Cooked halibut (3 ounces): 91 milligrams
- Almonds (1 ounce): 78 milligrams
- Peanut butter (2 tablespoons): 49 milligrams
- Spinach (2 cups): 47 milligrams
- Brown rice (½ cup): 42 milligrams.

FIBER

If you make one change from this book, let that be eating more fiber! Yes, we've talked about fiber before. Yes, we're talking about it again. Why? Improved digestion will improve your mood, and fiber is a big part of the digestive process, but it has other benefits like lowering cholesterol.

     ALL ABOUT FIBER

Here are more reasons that I LOVE fiber:

- Promotes a healthy weight
- Lowers blood pressure
- Lowers cholesterol
- Reduces the risk of heart disease
- Eases constipation
- Help control blood sugar
- Can reduce risk of certain cancers.

Most Americans don't get enough fiber, so aim for 14 grams of fiber for every 1,000 calories consumed.

Aim to include these fiber-rich foods in your diet several times a week. As a bonus, many of these foods provide other valuable nutrients, such as iron and potassium to your diet and are included in the recipes that you will find later in the book.

- Cooked black beans (½ cup): 7.7 grams
- Baked sweet potato, with peel: 4.8 grams
- Whole wheat English muffin: 4.4 grams
- 1 cup brown rice: 3.5 grams
- ½ cup cooked pasta: 2 grams
- 1 cup raisin bran cereal: 7.5 grams
- 1 apple: 3.5 grams
- Small pear: 4.4 grams.

Overall, when you look at the recommended foods from this list, you'll see they are mainly whole foods. They're less processed and the foods we all "know" we should be eating more of. I hope by seeing all the benefits of these foods, you'll take the time to shop in the produce section and incorporate these foods into your diet.

I also encourage you to aim for variety in your diet. It's okay to meal plan and rotate the same meals. However, I recommend you vary the types of protein and your fruits and veggies. Have black bean tacos one week, fish tacos the next, and use chicken the week after.

Variety is beneficial in your fruits and vegetables too. Pick produce that's in season. Typically, this will be less expensive and taste better. Think about how amazing a summer tomato or juicy June peach is! Choosing different fruits and vegetables will give you variety in your diet, which will give your body a variety of beneficial antioxidants too. That's why nutrition experts say to "eat the rainbow." When it comes to produce, the different colors are derived from different antioxidants that all have slightly different benefits to your body. Vary your produce, vary the colors, and I promise your body will thank you!

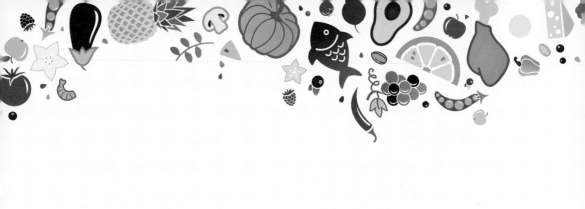

CHAPTER 6

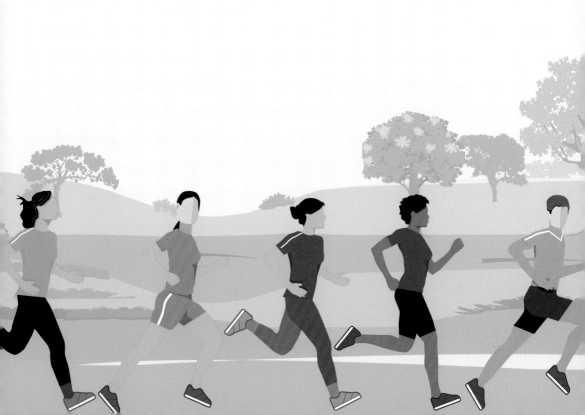

WEIGHT LOSS AND EXERCISE

How to lose weight without a crash diet!

Carissa Galloway, RDN

....

WEIGHT LOSS AND EXERCISE

Most of us have tried to diet and lose weight in the past. We've had some successes and I hope you've learned something from this book so far about which diets do and don't work for you. Have you dieted and lost weight and then regained it? That's frustrating, but unfortunately, that's the norm. Research says that most people gain back weight lost within 6 months. I don't say that to discourage you, I say that to make sure you understand why this book is education- and cognitive-based. Jeff and I want you to learn about nutrition, learn about what foods nourish your body, and learn how to activate your brain to make smart food choices that will support weight loss.

Weight loss happens in the kitchen. By creating a healthy calorie deficit. Once you reach your goal weight, exercise becomes equally important in the maintenance phase.

What does a healthy weight-loss program consist of?

- A reasonable, realistic weight-loss goal. No more than 10 pounds in 6 months.
- A reduced calorie, balanced eating plan.
- Regular physical exercise or increased physical exercise.
- A behavior change plan to help you stay on track with your goals.

Things to remember:

- Calories count. Yes, you should count them for the first month of a weight-loss program to understand your current diet and how food choices add up when it comes to calories.
- Portions count. Yes, you should measure them and read labels.
- Nutrition counts. Quality calorie vs empty calorie. You can gain weight from eating too many apples. You can gain weight from eating too many jellybeans. What food nourishes your body, provides antioxidants and fiber, and will actually fill you? Pick the apple over the jellybeans, and base your diet around whole foods with nutrition benefits.

- Even small weight loss can lead to big health benefits.
- Our goal is to develop good habits that last a lifetime.
- Discuss any major diet changes with your physician.

What does a successful weight-loss "loser" do?

- Commits to an exercise plan.
- Exercises for benefits outside of weight loss.
- Reduces calories, refined sugar, and saturated fat intake.
- Eats regular meals, including breakfast.
- Weighs themselves regularly. I recommend weekly, in the morning, on the same day each week.
- Doesn't let small "slips" turn into big rebound weight gain.

Now, I want you to read those bullet points again. Read them out loud.

When making your goals for weight loss keep these things in mind:

- Is your goal specific?
- Is your goal measurable?
- Does your goal have a specific timeline of fewer than 6 months in which it can be achieved?
- Can I get feedback on my progress toward this goal?

Now I want you to pause and think about your weight-loss goals. Visualize yourself reaching those goals. Even better if you write down your goals. Write them in the book, write them in a journal, write them in the notes section of your phone. When you put goals in writing they become a road map to progress. Defining your goals is an important step on any weight-loss journey.

HOW MANY CALORIES DO I NEED PER DAY?

Starting a cognitive-focused weight-loss plan means having a range of calories you are striving for. Without fancy machines, it can be a challenge to find your EXACT daily caloric needs but having a goal will give you something to strive for.

Eating too many calories leads to weight gain. BUT eating too few calories can also lead to weight gain. This is because when you consistently give your body a caloric intake below its needs, your body thinks it is starving. When our body is "starving," it will store calories/energy/fat. We don't want this. Finding a baseline calorie goal will give us something to strive for so we don't eat too many or too few calories.

Our basal metabolic rate or our baseline calorie needs are influenced by many things, including age, sex, ethnicity, exercise level, current weight, medication. You and your sister may have a similar weight; however, you could have calorie needs that vary by up to 500 calories per day.

Here is a very simplistic calorie formula for weight loss. This one does not consider age, activity, or gender, but it is very straightforward in its design.

1. Current Weight (in pounds) × 11 = Caloric Baseline
2. Caloric Baseline + 400 = Daily Caloric Needs
3. Daily Caloric Need - 500 calories = Estimated Daily Calories for Weight Loss.

As a note, I don't recommend anyone ever dipping below 1,200 calories a day. This is too low and will often lead to binging and weight regain.

Once you find your calorie goal, you can use a calorie- and meal-tracking app to see how many calories you should aim to eat in a day. Strive for the caloric goal you found above and see how your body responds. You may need to alter your caloric goal for weight loss and that's okay. Make small tweaks until you see progress on the scale.

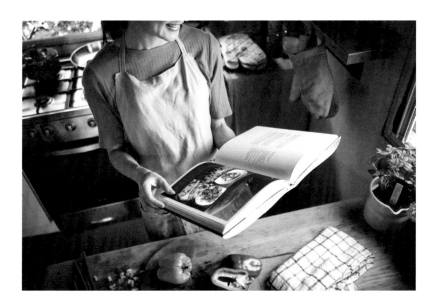

BLUEPRINT FOR WEIGHT-LOSS SUCCESS

- Eat 4 to 5 small meals a day
- Eat every 3 to 4 hours
- Eat clean, unprocessed foods
- Eat protein and fiber with every meal/snack.

Remember the three Ps
1. **Prepare.** Plan what you're going to eat. Pack food and snacks wherever you go. Prepare meals ahead of time. Look at menus and nutrition facts before you go out to restaurants. If you have a game plan, you are more likely to make the right food decisions and less likely to make bad, emotional eating decisions.
2. **Portion.** Pay attention to how much you eat. Measure your food when you eat at home and eat half of restaurant portions, saving the rest for another meal.
3. **Protein.** Eat some type of protein with every meal or snack. There's a lot of science behind this one. Some of the benefits of consuming protein include a satiety boost, meaning you feel full. There's also the thermic effect of protein digestion, which means that it takes your body calories to digest and then utilize the protein you consume. Aim never to eat carbs alone . . . pair them with protein!

SAMPLE DAILY EATING SCHEDULE

8 a.m. Breakfast
10:30 a.m. Snack
1 p.m. Lunch
4 p.m. Snack 2
7 p.m. Dinner
These times are approximate, but I wanted to show you how to fuel your body. It will feel like you're always eating. That's a GOOD thing because it keeps your metabolic fire burning and thus your body burning calories.

Breakfast Options (pick one):

- ½ cup oatmeal (not instant) with 8 ounces milk of your choice, 1 ounce nuts, and ¼ cup dried fruit or ½ cup fresh fruit
- 3 egg whites with 2 pieces of whole grain toast; you can add veggies and salsa to the eggs
- Greek yogurt and a banana

- 1 cup high-fiber cereal with 8 ounces milk of your choice and ½ cup berries
- ½ 100-percent whole wheat bagel with peanut butter
- Protein pancake
- Smoothie made with 1 scoop whey protein, ½ cup strawberries (or any fruit), and milk of your choice
- A note on milks: I prefer you choose a milk with protein.

My tip: Breakfast is the easiest meal of the day to do right! Pick well and measure your portions!

Morning Snack Options (pick one):

- 1 green apple with 2 tablespoons of natural peanut butter
- ½ cup cottage cheese and pineapple
- 200 calorie or less protein bar
- Greek yogurt
- Nut bar with at least 4 grams of fiber and 6 grams of protein
- Ready-to-drink protein shake
- Any of the afternoon snack options.

Always have healthy snacks at work, in your car, and purse. I never leave the house without a protein bar, apple, and huge bottle of water.

Lunch Options (pick one):

- 3 ounces sliced turkey, 2 slices of whole grain bread, and a side salad with a vinegar-based dressing
- 4 ounces grilled chicken, a medium-sized baked sweet potato, and 1 cup of green beans, zucchini, and any green vegetable
- 3 ounces canned tuna mixed with 1 tablespoon of low-fat mayo and 6 light crackers
- 4 ounces chicken wrapped in a whole wheat tortilla with salsa and 1 ounce cheddar cheese and ½ cup black beans
- Sushi like a brown rice California roll, salmon roll, tuna roll, or vegetable roll
- Turkey burger or veggie burger on a whole grain roll
- Use your healthy leftovers from last night!
- Frozen meal with less than 450 calories and at least 10 grams of protein.

My tip is to use your leftovers from the day before. This way you've PLANNED and know you have a healthy option.

Afternoon Snack Options (pick one):

- 1 slice of whole wheat bread, 1 tablespoon peanut butter, 1 teaspoon natural jelly (limit peanut butter to one serving daily)
- Protein shake and an orange
- 6 ounces low-fat yogurt and 12 almonds (or walnuts—get dry roasted)
- Hummus with any carrots, celery, bell pepper
- Low-fat string cheese, small apple, and 6 whole wheat crackers
- 3 ounces low-sodium deli turkey or chicken breast, 6 whole wheat crackers, 1 wedge laughing cow cheese.

I try to have an apple on an empty stomach every day. This adds a fiber boost and supports healthy digestion. Why do I choose to have it on an empty stomach? A wise nutrition professor in college explained it this way. It made perfect sense, and I've committed to it ever since. She said to think about the insoluble fiber in the apple as a toothbrush. When you eat the apple, it has to ability to work through your digestion and clean up things along the way. Eating it on an empty stomach or between meals allows it to be most effective. Think of the difference between brushing your teeth five minutes after eating or five hours after eating. The apple cleans your digestive tract which in turn supports digestion and can reduce bloating.

Dinner Options (pick one):

- 4 ounces any white fish (grilled or baked) with ½ cup black beans and ½ cup brown rice; use lemon to season
- 4 ounces grilled chicken and 1 medium-sized baked sweet potato and 1 cup steamed asparagus
- 4 ounces lean ground turkey breast and ½ cup whole wheat penne pasta, ½ cup marinara sauce, and a spinach salad with a vinaigrette dressing
- 4 ounces ginger chicken stir-fried with 1 cup broccoli and carrots and ½ cup brown rice.

Limit eating after dinner and don't eat after 8 p.m.! If hungry, drink water or a hot tea or if necessary, have a protein shake!

Drinks:

- Drink A LOT of water! This is so important!
- You can have coffee in the morning and all the unsweetened tea and sparkling water you want.
- Avoid diet sodas and alcohol . . . please!

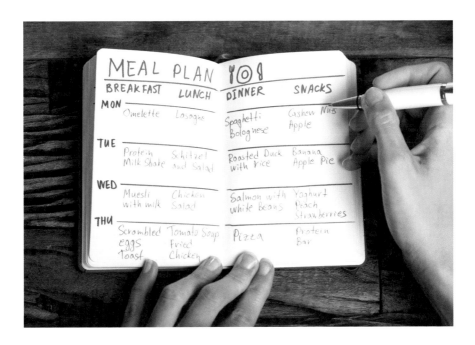

MEAL PLANNING

I am a HUGE fan of meal planning. My clients that are the most successful in maintaining weight loss commit to meal planning and most of them also devote time to meal prep. That time in thoughtful prep pays huge dividends in making healthier, more balanced food choices. My goal is that in time, you can write your own meal plans like the ones later in this book, even if they are very simplistic.

Here's an example of my dinner plans for a typical week:

Monday—roasted salmon with asparagus and microwave rice (can sub chicken or other white fish)

Tuesday—slow cooker vegetarian chili

Wednesday—garlic dill salmon with baked potatoes

Thursday—vegetarian meatballs with zucchini and pesto

Friday—take-out Indian.

Breakfast rotates between oatmeal and toast with either peanut butter or avocado and both with a serving of fruit. Lunch is leftovers because I always make extra dinner or a fiber- and protein-rich vegetarian frozen meal.

HEALTHY SWAPS

Weight loss doesn't need to be cumbersome. Simple swaps can add up to a calorie deficit that over the course of a few months, can help your body maintain an ideal weight. When you're looking to upgrade your diet and lower your daily caloric intake in the process, try these smart swaps.

Remember, at its core, weight loss is a numbers game, so cutting 50 calories a day can add up to a decrease of 18,250 calories a year, which would equal about 5 pounds lost from just a small change!

- Swap potato chips for pistachios
  - » Pistachios can give crunch, and there are plenty of flavored options available, such as chili roasted. Pistachios give you a trio of plant-based protein, fiber, and better-for-you mono- and polyunsaturated fats, which potato chips don't have. If you opt for in-shell pistachios, then taking the time to crack the shells will slow down your snacking and thus you end up eating less.
- Swap a candy bar for a chocolate protein shake
  - » You will get the chocolate you crave with either option; however, your blood sugar will thank you for picking the satiety-boosting 30 grams of protein in the Premier Protein shake, plus it's just 160 calories with 1 gram of sugar, 24 vitamins and minerals and antioxidants, and vitamins C and E to help support a healthy immune system. Plus, since there's only 1 gram of sugar in the Premier Protein shake, that's a big improvement over the almost 29 grams of sugar in a Snickers bar.
- Swap movie theater-style popcorn for air popped popcorn at home
  - » Popcorn is a whole grain, so there are benefits to keeping it in your diet. Aim to use no oil on the stovetop, but if you do, pick an oil with a higher smoke point, such as walnut or avocado.
- Swap a Reese's Peanut Butter Cup for a DIY peanut butter-filled date
  - » To make them, add a slit in the middle of your date and remove the pit. Fill with ½ teaspoon natural peanut butter and enjoy. You could also dip them in melted chocolate for the full Reese's experience. Dates are packed with antioxidants, fiber, and have no added sugar.

- Can you make a swap for ice cream?
  - » Not many things will give you that creamy texture of ice cream. You can try frozen yogurt or the many lower calorie options available in the grocery store. Two other options that I've found success with my clients are berries with whipped cream and banana ice cream. Berries with whipped cream give you the creaminess of ice cream and the vitamins, minerals, and fiber in the berries. Banana ice cream is more time consuming to make, but provides a great texture with a boost of potassium and no added sugar. To make banana ice cream, use only frozen bananas and combine one or two with 1 tablespoon of milk per banana and pulse in a food processor until you reach your desired consistency. Top with shredded coconut or a few mini chocolate morsels.
- Swap your pretzels for lentil chips
  - » Pretzels are less saturated fat than other salty snacks like chips, but they are mainly refined carbohydrates and salt, and unless you pair them with a dip like hummus, they don't have much staying power. Lentil chips will give you a crunch with a large serving size and more protein than pretzels.
- Two swaps for your fries—and they're both best in the air fryer
  - » My family makes air fryer fries all the time and they're delish! The key is to soak your potato after cutting for 20 minutes. This draws out the starch and makes the fries extra crisp. You won't miss the oil! I also like using zucchini as a substitute for fries. My recipe has parmesan in the breading for extra flavor. Even if you actually fry them (I recommend air fryer or baking), you'll have less carbohydrates and more fiber than a potato.
- Keep the nachos and swap the chip base
  - » Use roasted sweet potato rounds as the "chips" and focus on vegetables and fiber in your toppings, such as black beans, bell peppers, corn, fresh tomatoes, and avocado. Sweet potatoes are a good source of fiber, fat-free, and packed with vitamins A, C, B6, E, and potassium. To keep it healthier, limit fat and extra calories by exchanging sour cream for a flavor-packed cheese like queso fresco after broiling the nachos. A small bit of this crumbly cheese will add great flavor.
- Swap soda for less soda and MORE ice
  - » Soda is something that I 100 percent recommend my clients cut out of their daily diet. I'm not a big fan of diet soda either, and through years in practice, I know cutting out soda is HARD. Start by diluting your soda. Fill a cup with as much ice as possible and pour half the soda you would usually consume in the glass. The ice will melt and dilute your soda so you will be minimizing the calories and extra added sugar just a little bit

(and boosting hydration because ice is water when it melts!). Over time, I recommend completely cutting out soda from your diet. Another option is flavored seltzer waters. The bubbles are still there and the flavors are more interesting than plain water.

Weight-loss "rules" that work:

- Eat more vegetables
  - » Filling half your plate with vegetables will help you feel full and allow you to eat fewer calories.
- Drink more water
  - » Drinking water allows you to avoid extra liquid calories.
  - » The average American drinks 245 calories per day. That's 90,000 calories a year and 26 pounds!
- Table, chair, plate
  - » Don't even think about eating without sitting at a table, in a chair and eating off a plate. This prevents mindless eating and allows you to experience your food. You are more likely to enjoy the meal and be satisfied by eating less.
- The apple rule
  - » Next time you mindlessly walk into the kitchen looking for a snack, try to ask yourself if you are really hungry or just eating out of habit or boredom?
  - » If you're really hungry, you would eat an apple. If you wouldn't, then look to why else you might want to eat.
- Eat cereal for breakfast
  - » Studies show that people who eat cereal for breakfast 5 days a week weigh less than those who don't, have a lower risk of diabetes, and consume more fiber and calcium.
  - » Good choices include: oatmeal, Kashi cereals, Total, or Grape Nuts.
- The kitchen is closed
  - » Close your kitchen for 12 hours each day.
  - » Studies show that late night snacking can significantly increase your weight and lead to 31 extra pounds a year.
  - » This can also be a form of intermittent fasting. Aim for a 12-hour circadian fast, closing the kitchen after your evening meal and not opening the kitchen until 12 hours after that evening meal.
- Eat at home
  - » Aim to eat 90 percent of meals at home . . . yes 90 percent.

» Restaurant portions are larger, have more fat and sodium than you would eat at home. Over time, this can lead to weight gain if you constantly choose restaurant food over cooking at home.
- Move more
  » Weight loss is NOT just diet. You need to burn more calories by exercising.
  » Try 10 minutes a day walking up and down stairs, and research says you'll lose 10 pounds a year.
  » Workout for 45 minutes instead of 30, and you could lose 30 extra pounds a year.

WEIGHT-LOSS PLATEAU

One of the most frustrating parts of being on any weight-loss journey is seeing results stop—the dreaded plateau. First of all, if you are experiencing a plateau, don't let that make you stop trying! Plateaus are the point where many people stop and lose all the progress and cognitive strategies that have supported the change this far.

Why does your body do this to you?

During the first few weeks of losing weight, a rapid drop is normal. In part, this is because when you cut calories, the body gets needed energy initially by releasing its stores of glycogen, a type of carbohydrate found in the muscles and liver.

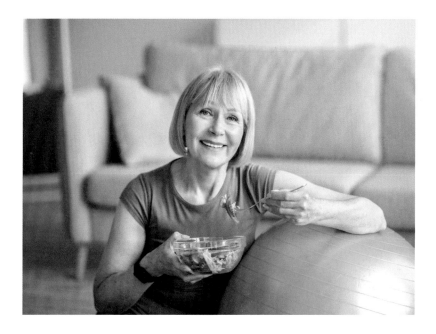

Glycogen is partly made of water, so when glycogen is burned for energy, it releases water, resulting in weight loss that's mostly water. This effect is temporary, however.

As you lose weight, you lose some muscle along with fat. Muscle helps keep the rate at which you burn calories (metabolism) up. As you lose weight, your metabolism declines, causing you to burn fewer calories than you did at your heavier weight.

Your slower metabolism will slow your weight loss, even if you eat the same number of calories that helped you lose weight. When the calories you burn equal the calories you eat, you reach a plateau.

To lose more weight, you need to either increase your physical activity or decrease the calories you eat. Using the same approach that worked initially may maintain your weight loss, but it won't lead to more weight loss.

Tips for when you encounter a plateau:

- Go back to logging. Look for patterns and changes from when you were first successful.
- Take stock of your current lifestyle. Have there been any major changes to your activity level, sleep, or stress? If so, try to shift those back to when you saw results.
- Adjust your current calorie intake—as you lose weight, your body needs a different number of daily calories. Use the formulas from the beginning of the program to calculate your calories at your new weight.
- What are you eating? Focus on quality, whole foods and avoid processed or "grab and go" foods.
- Beware of nibbles. Are you the cook or do you have kids? Cooking and feeding kids can add in daily "nibbles." Testing a meal's seasoning or grabbing a bite off your kids' unfinished plates. All those nibbles or cleaning up kids' plates add up and probably don't make it into your log. I had a nutrition professor tell me that a "nibbler" may add up to 200 calories a day, which as a big "Aha!" moment for me when it comes to the impact of small, mindless bites.
- Cut liquid calories. Weekend wine? Midday latte? For 2 weeks, work hard to eliminate those and see how the scale responds.
- Strength train. As you build muscle, you are burning calories and creating a more metabolically active body.

- Eat more protein. Protein has the highest thermic effect of food, meaning eating protein burns more calories during digestion. Protein also contains an amino acid, leucine, which numerous research studies have identified as a potent catalyst for burning body fat.
- Move more! Weight loss is an equation. You need to burn more than you take in from food, and moving more is the key to keeping weight off. Add in more daily movement by taking the stairs, parking farther away, or committing to an evening walk. Also, make it a goal to exercise for at least 30 minutes at least 3 days a week. Alternate what type of exercise you do and vary the intensity to get the most benefits.

SLEEP AND WEIGHT LOSS

Food and exercise will impact your health and your weight. If you are aiming to lose weight, I encourage you to look closely at your sleep habits. Why? Research found that for every hour less of sleep during a week, people ate 210 more calories, mainly from fat and carbohydrates. Read that again . . . less sleep can lead to your brain telling you to eat more, and those cravings aren't your fault. When your body is tired, it seeks to "fix" that with a quick boost from sugar or fats.

Lack of sleep can cause a negative cycle that leads to weight gain. When you're sleep deprived, your body increases its hunger cravings. These cravings cause you to eat more, as mentioned previously, and the increased caloric intake leads to weight gain. If weight gain continues, it can cause other sleep issues, such as sleep apnea or insomnia. If you continue to be sleep deprived, your body will continue to crave sugar and fats, and you could continue to gain weight.

It's hard to simply say "get more sleep." I know it can be a challenge, and I don't claim to be a sleep expert. What helps our family is regular exercise, not having a television in the bedroom, using a white noise machine, and using a mediation app before bed. Aim for 7 to 8 hours of sleep per day.

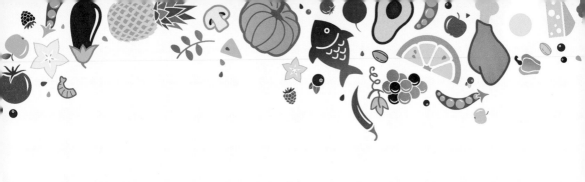

CHAPTER 7

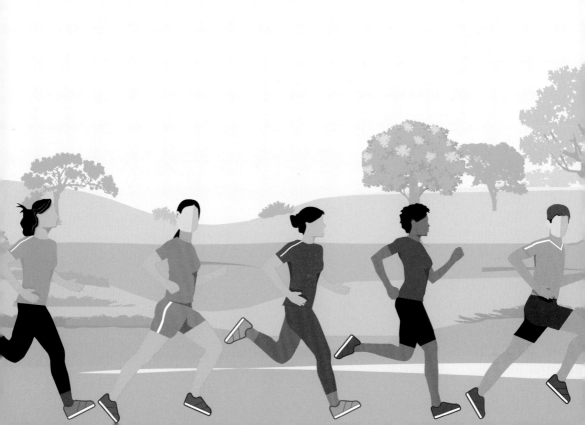

MEAL PLANS AND MEAL PREP

If you want to run a marathon, you have a training plan. When weight loss is your goal, it's the same—start here with a meal plan!

Carissa Galloway, RDN

When people learn that I'm a dietitian, their first questions are usually about weight loss. What do I recommend, and how to lose weight quickly? People want an easy solution and a quick fix. They usually also want a meal plan. I hesitate to hand out meal plans to someone unless I know they're serious about weight loss. The reason why is that a meal plan without education on nutrition will only work for so long. That's why we're at chapter 7 and I'm only now sharing meal plans. I want you to have already established not only nutrition knowledge but also knowledge about your current diet and caloric intake level. Once you have that knowledge, meal plans are simply a guide to implementing other strategies we've talked about. It's just a tool and not a magic wand. You already know you must do the work, and the meal plan is here to help you get started.

 MORE MEAL PREP ADVICE

SAMPLE MEAL PLANS

Following are two sample meal plans with grocery lists. When your motivation is at its highest to lose weight, I highly recommend you dive into these meal plans. They will give you structure to balance your diet and start a pattern of cooking at home. You can adjust the proteins or vegetables to fit your taste preferences. You can also adjust the portions to fit your caloric goal for weight loss.

Week 1 Meal Plan

MEAL	BREAKFAST	SNACK	LUNCH	SNACK	DINNER
MONDAY	Homemade egg sandwich with 2 eggs, spinach, ¼ avocado, whole wheat English muffin 1 cup berries	Small fruit (apple, orange, pear) 1 mozzarella string cheese	Homemade tuna salad with whole wheat pita and crudité	Celery sticks Natural PB	Baked or grilled fish or chicken (cook extra chicken or fish for lunches) Roasted asparagus ½ cup brown rice
TUESDAY	¾ cup old-fashioned oats (not instant) with 1 tablespoon honey Berries 1 tablespoon nut butter	Apple + 1 tablespoon nut butter	½ cup brown rice 4 oz chicken breast or fish (cooked on Monday p.m.) Raw bell peppers	1 cup steamed edamame in pods	Ground turkey 1 cup zucchini Marinara sauce (cook extra turkey and zucchini for lunches)
WEDNESDAY	Homemade egg sandwich with 2 eggs, spinach, ¼ avocado, whole wheat English muffin 1 cup berries	Small fruit (apple, orange, pear) 1 mozzarella string cheese	½ cup whole wheat pasta Ground turkey (cooked on Tuesday p.m.) Marinara sauce	Celery sticks Natural PB	Baked pesto salmon with broccoli ½ cup basmati rice (cook extra salmon for lunches)
THURSDAY	¾ cup old-fashioned oats (not instant) cooked with milk or milk alternative with at least 7 grams of protein 1 banana	4, 3-inch dried mango strips 49 pistachios	½ cup whole wheat pasta Ground turkey (cooked on Tuesday p.m.) Marinara sauce	3 slices low-sodium turkey, 6 crackers, small low-sodium V8	Slow cooker BBQ chicken sliders, whole wheat pita, and coleslaw

MEAL	BREAKFAST	SNACK	LUNCH	SNACK	DINNER
FRIDAY	High-protein cereal (at least 7 grams of protein) with milk or milk alternative Fruit	Small fruit (apple, orange, pear) 1 mozzarella string cheese	Leftover salmon pesto basmati rice bowl (cooked on Wednesday p.m.)	1 cup steamed edamame in pods	Meal Out: Chipotle chicken bowl with only chicken, veggies, and pico de gallo or similar. Focus on protein and veggies and if you can save some for lunch tomorrow, do that!
SATURDAY	Pumpkin-baked oatmeal ½ cup berries	4, 3-inch dried mango strips 49 pistachios	Homemade tuna salad with whole wheat pita and crudité	3 slices low-sodium turkey, 6 crackers, small low-sodium V8	Dinner Out No carbs or cheese. Save ½ of meal as leftovers for lunch if possible
SUNDAY	Brunch out OR pumpkin-baked oatmeal ½ cup berries	Apple + 1 tablespoon nut butter	Leftovers from the week	1 mozzarella string cheese, celery sticks	Ground beef or turkey Oven-baked tacos with black beans, peppers, and onions (cook extra tacos for lunches)

Week 2 Meal Plan

MEAL	BREAKFAST	SNACK	LUNCH	SNACK	DINNER
MONDAY	Purple pomegranate juice smoothie Whole wheat toast with nut butter	4 ounces cottage cheese topped with peach or canned peaches in juice	Leftover oven baked tacos from Sunday night	High-fiber granola or nut bar 12 grapes	Italian chicken with vegetables (cook extra for lunches) Roasted red potatoes
TUESDAY	Leftover pumpkin-baked oatmeal Diced pear	Apple + 1 tablespoon nut butter	Amy's Organic Frozen Meal	Carrot sticks, sliced cucumber 4 ounces natural beef or turkey jerky	Mexican black bean and rice bowl with guacamole Romaine salad (cook extra for lunches)
WEDNESDAY	Purple pomegranate juice smoothie Whole wheat toast with nut butter	High-fiber granola or nut bar 12 grapes	Leftover Italian chicken with vegetables Whole wheat pita toasted and topped with parmesan cheese	Celery sticks Natural PB	Almond-crusted tilapia with green beans (cook extra for lunches) Roasted red potatoes
THURSDAY	2 scrambled eggs with spinach, avocado, and whole wheat toast	4 ounces cottage cheese topped with peach or canned peaches in juice	Mexican black bean and rice bowl with guacamole	High-fiber granola or nut bar 12 grapes	Grilled cumin chicken with mango salsa, salad, and rice (can substitute shrimp for chicken or use black beans to make it a vegetarian dinner)

MEAL	BREAKFAST	SNACK	LUNCH	SNACK	DINNER
FRIDAY	High-protein cereal (at least 7 grams of protein) with milk or milk alternative Fruit	Small fruit (apple, orange, pear) 49 pistachios	Leftover tilapia with rice	Carrot sticks, sliced cucumber 4 ounces natural beef or turkey jerky	Meal Out: Focus on protein and veggies, and if you can save some for lunch tomorrow, do that!
SATURDAY	Hash brown egg nests (make extra for next week) Berries	4 ounces cottage cheese topped with peach or canned peaches in juice	Amy's Organic Frozen Meal	Celery sticks Natural PB	Taco salad using extra grilled cumin chicken or any grilled fish
SUNDAY	Brunch out OR Pumpkin-baked oatmeal ½ cup berries	Apple + 1 tablespoon nut butter	Leftovers from the week	Carrot sticks, sliced cucumber 4 ounces natural beef or turkey jerky	Skinny turkey lasagna

GROCERY LIST FOR MEAL PLAN ONE

- ◯ Dozen eggs
- ◯ 1 avocado
- ◯ 1 container organic spinach
- ◯ Whole wheat English muffins
- ◯ 2 containers of berries: raspberries, blackberries, blueberries, strawberries, pineberries
- ◯ 4 apples
- ◯ 3 mozzarella string cheese
- ◯ Old Fashioned Oats
- ◯ Honey
- ◯ 1 container nut butter of choice
- ◯ Milk or milk alternative with at least 7 grams of protein per serving
- ◯ High-protein cereal like Kashi with at least 7 grams of protein per serving
- ◯ 1 can of pure pumpkin
- ◯ 1 package dried mango
- ◯ 1 package pistachios
- ◯ 2 cans of tuna
- ◯ 3 whole wheat pitas
- ◯ Baby carrots
- ◯ Celery
- ◯ 2 red or yellow bell peppers
- ◯ 1 white onion
- ◯ 2 packages chicken breast
- ◯ Asparagus
- ◯ 2 zucchinis
- ◯ 2 microwaveable brown rice packages brown rice packages
- ◯ Frozen edamame in pods
- ◯ 1 package lean ground turkey breast (or lean ground grass-fed beef or Impossible/Beyond Burger)
- ◯ 1 jar marinara sauce
- ◯ BBQ sauce
- ◯ Coleslaw
- ◯ 6 ounces low-sodium turkey slices
- ◯ 1 box wheat thins
- ◯ Low-sodium V8
- ◯ 1 can black beans
- ◯ Whole wheat tortillas
- ◯ Whole wheat pasta (penne preferred)

GROCERY LIST FOR MEAL PLAN TWO

- ○ Pomegranate juice
- ○ 3 bananas
- ○ Yogurt for smoothie
- ○ Milk or non-dairy milk for smoothie
- ○ Spinach for smoothie
- ○ Whole grain/whole wheat toast
- ○ Nut butter
- ○ Pear
- ○ Berries
- ○ Dozen eggs
- ○ Spinach
- ○ 2 avocados
- ○ High-protein cereal with at least 7 grams of protein
- ○ Salsa
- ○ Refrigerated hash brown potatoes
- ○ Cheddar cheese
- ○ 3 × 4-ounce containers for cottage cheese
- ○ 3 peaches or 3 containers of peaches canned in juice
- ○ 3 high-fiber or nut bars like KIND or Lärabars
- ○ 1 package grapes
- ○ 3 apples
- ○ 2 frozen meals with at least 9 grams of protein, 5 grams of fiber, less than 450 mg of sodium. I prefer the Amy's Organic brand.
- ○ 2 cans of black beans
- ○ 2 packages of microwaveable brown rice packages
- ○ 1 container of guacamole
- ○ Carrot sticks
- ○ Celery sticks
- ○ Nitrate-free beef or turkey jerky
- ○ 2 to 3 packages of chicken breast
- ○ 1 bag of red potatoes
- ○ Extra virgin olive oil
- ○ 1 bottle Greek salad dressing
- ○ 2 zucchinis
- ○ Asparagus
- ○ 2 bags of romaine lettuce
- ○ 1 cucumber

- Mango salsa
- No-bake lasagna noodles
- 16 oz ricotta cheese
- 1 package ground turkey
- Parsley
- 1 container marinara sauce

I like meal plans because, just like training plans that Jeff makes for running, they give you a guide—a place to start as you work toward making positive changes in your nutrition routine. I also highly recommend that you give these two meal plans a try and then write your own.

Yes, you become the dietitian and write down a 1-week meal plan that fits your lifestyle and food preferences. Use these meal plans as a guide but add in family favorite meals. Then whenever you feel like your diet has "gone off track," you can come back to your self-created meal plan and get your focus back!

Your kitchen tells the future, so always have it stocked to make better-for-you meals easier.

A well-stocked kitchen has:

- Veggies—especially quick cook ones and leafy greens
- Frozen veggies for quick side dishes
- Fruit—vary colors for added nutrients
- Lean meats
- Seafood—canned and frozen for quick meals
- Whole grains—breads, rice, whole grain pasta
- Beans
- Nuts
- Eggs

THE PICK THREE PLAN

Even with the best intentions, it can be a challenge to get all the variety in each meal that your body needs for optimal nutrition. If I was creating a perfect meal or snack it would include:

- Complex carbohydrate
- Lean protein
- A source of healthy fats
- Produce (fruit or vegetable) and
- A source of fiber.

When you plan a meal or snack aim to include at least three of the previously listed foods.

When you start building your own meals, start with this rule of three. This will allow you to improve the quality of your diet and create more balance in your meals without feeling like you must be "perfect" to achieve success.

Here are some examples of meals and snacks made with the "pick three plan."

Whole grain toast with peanut butter and sliced strawberries
- Complex carbohydrate and fiber—whole grain toast
- Healthy fat and protein source—peanut butter
- Produce—strawberries.

Bean chili with a baked potato topped with avocado
- Complex carbohydrate and fiber—beans
- Carbohydrate—potato
- Protein source—beans
- Healthy fat—avocado
- Produce—tomato and other vegetables used in chili cooking.

Whole wheat pasta with turkey meatballs in marinara sauce and roasted broccoli
- Complex carbohydrate—pasta
- Protein source—turkey
- Produce—broccoli, tomatoes in marinara sauce
- If you added flax seeds to a turkey meatball blend, you could add a healthy fat.

Greek yogurt parfait
- Carbohydrate and protein—yogurt (remember milk contains lactose, which is a milk sugar and, as such, a carbohydrate)
- Healthy fat and protein source—chopped walnuts
- Produce—any fruit used to top the yogurt.

Hummus with carrot sticks and six whole grain crackers
- Complex carbohydrate—crackers
- Healthy fat and protein source—hummus
- Produce—carrots.

Greek salad with chicken and chickpeas
- Carbohydrate and fiber—chickpeas
- Healthy fat—olive oil used in dressing
- Protein source—chicken
- Produce—whatever you use in the salad: spinach, tomatoes, cucumber, bell pepper.

MEAL PREP

What does "meal prep" mean? It simply means planning and even preparing some of your meals ahead of time. Instead of walking through the door exhausted after work and wondering what's for dinner, you walk in the door knowing what's for dinner and, since you cooked part of it the night before, then your dinner is ready in less time!

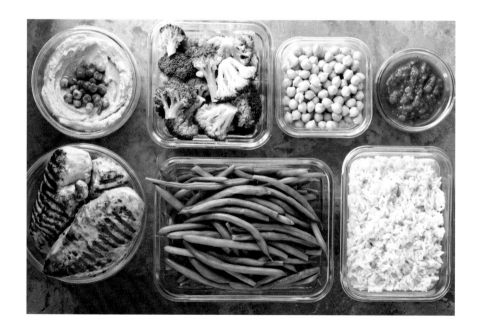

I am a HUGE advocate for meal planning and meal prep, and I'm not alone in this. Research continually shows that those who make time for meal planning and meal prep not only eat a healthier, more balanced diet, but because they choose take-out foods less often, they tend to weigh less. Research shows that spending more time on food preparation is directly linked to increased vegetable, fruit, and salad consumption.

BENEFITS OF MEAL PREP

- Improved quality of your diet
- Improved variety in your diet
- Linked to weight loss and obesity prevention
  - » People who don't meal prep eat more meals out or get more take-out. The more meals you eat out or get as take-out leads to consuming more fat, sodium, and large portions. Just by swapping this for meals made at home, can help you lose weight.
- Saves money
  - » The cost of food and eating out has been increasing steadily, and you can save significantly if you cook at home. A salad at a quick service restaurant can cost around $12. To make one quickly at home, buy a rotisserie chicken ($8), a bagged salad ($4), and an avocado to add some nutrients ($2). That's a total of $14. However, you can feed at least two people with the salad, and you can use the leftover rotisserie chicken and avocado for a quick taco for lunch the next day. Just add tortillas, cheese, and some salsa!
- Saves time
  - » It may seem counterintuitive, but meal prepping and cooking at home saves time. Most people choose take-out because it's faster; however, with time and routine, cooking at home can become faster and provide you with nutritious food in less time. Think about how easy it is to simply heat up leftovers! Make a large batch of pasta and roasted vegetables on Monday and enjoy them for lunch again on Tuesday with less than 5 minutes to heat them up.
- May help you live longer
  - » Research has found that eating more meals away from home is significantly associated with increased risk of death by any cause. In one study, individuals who ate at home often (meaning they had less than one take-out meal per week) lived longer than those who dined out frequently (those who dined out two meals or more per day).
- Reduces food waste
  - » This is a book about nutrition and not a book about saving the planet; however, we all waste far too much food. We throw out food when portions are too big. We throw out food that spoils. We throw out less food when

we meal prep and plan because we are more focused at the store and shop smarter using what we buy.

» Cutting and prepping fruit and vegetables also makes you more likely to eat them, and they are less likely to spoil and be thrown out.

• Improved emotional wellness

» It can be stressful coming home after a long day and contemplating what's for dinner. Meal prep answers that question. The meal is already decided. Imagine the huge sigh of relief that would bring. Your planning ahead gives you less stress in a hectic moment.

» There is limited research on meal prep and emotional health. However, one study observed a significant association between time spent on daily meal prep and higher self-rated mental health, as well as lower self-rated stress. Further research suggests that when the burden of choice is removed from eating, the food relieves anxiety and anger and reduces systolic blood pressure, more than when a choice is involved. Make your choices when you meal plan weekly and then you won't have the daily "what's for dinner?" anxiety or question. Food becomes less of a burden and your emotional wellness improves.

HOW TO START MEAL PREPPING

You can start meal prepping and planning with just 10 minutes a week. Start with the two meal plans provided at the beginning of this chapter. On week three, sit down and think through your meals for the coming week. This is best done before you go to the grocery store and then you're stocking your kitchen for success again. I encourage you to plan out dinners first and then see what dinners you can work into lunches for other days of the week. This saves on time in the kitchen, makes more healthy choices available, and reduces food waste. Repeating meals is okay. You don't need to have the most creative kitchen. If any of the meals from the meal plan worked well for you, add those in, and build the rest of your meal plan with other family favorite meals. Consistency is key. Make a date with meal planning and, over time, you will refine your meal planning and the benefits will continue to grow.

WHERE TO FIND MEAL PREP IDEAS

When it comes to nutrition, I rarely recommend you turn to social media for advice. It's hard to police what's evidence-based nutrition, what's a fad diet that will backfire, and what's someone trying to make a buck by selling you a quick solution. However, I do find that social media is a great source of meal ideas. Seeing what someone eats or prepares can give you an "Aha!" moment of how to incorporate something new into your diet. I've found a lot of great meal prep ideas from bloggers and other dietitians.

Find them on social media, fill your feed with them, and then make the ideas your own. Some ideas that I've "borrowed" from social media include oven-baked burgers, air fryer cauliflower nuggets, and sheet pan meals galore.

SIMPLE IDEAS FOR MEAL PREP

- Cook extra—if you're taking the time to cook, then cook extra. Once the oven or grill is preheated, use that time and cooking energy to cook more. You will be amazed how helpful the leftovers can be.
  » Grill extra chicken, burgers, or fish
  » Roast extra vegetables. We love roasted broccoli, asparagus, and cauliflower
  » Cook extra grains. Extra rice or quinoa is wonderful to use in one-pot-recipes.
  » Cut fruits and vegetables when you get home from the store, and keep them at eye level.
- Rotisserie Chicken—rotisserie chicken is an easy, pre-cooked food that's perfect for a quick weeknight dinner and great in a variety of leftover dishes. Typically, protein is the part of the meal that takes the longest to cook.
  » Rotisserie chicken salad using a bagged salad kit. Add rice to boost carbs for training.
  » Rotisserie chicken breast with mashed potatoes and roasted vegetables.
  » Rotisserie chicken enchiladas.
  » BBQ rotisserie chicken flatbreads.
  » Rotisserie chicken fried rice.
  » Rotisserie chicken caprese panini.
- Pulled Pork—cook a pork shoulder in the Crock-Pot until it shreds easily. You can then use the pulled pork for several recipes throughout the week. Many of the rotisserie chicken ideas work with pulled pork too.
  » Green chile pork enchiladas with black beans.
  » Pulled pork nachos.
  » Loaded BBQ baked potato with pulled pork.
  » Pulled pork quesadilla.
  » Pulled pork sandwich with coleslaw.
  » Pulled pork "pizza" with BBQ sauce and cheddar on mini naan flatbreads.
- Bake meatballs—meatballs can work in many different dishes. Bake plain meatballs and you can serve them with pasta, as a sandwich, or my favorite with buffalo dipping sauce.
- Cook and peel hard-boiled eggs.
- Bake egg muffins.
- Make oatmeal-based fruit muffins.

- Place meat in marinades when you get home from the store and freeze so your meat is flavorful and ready to cook.
- Freeze fruit that's about to "expire" for quick smoothies. Add the fruit and spinach to a Ziploc bag, and when you need a smoothie, just combine frozen fruits and milk of your choice and other add-ins.
- Make pasta salad with pre-cooked pasta, leftover carrots, and tomato. Add Italian dressing and leftover grilled chicken for a quick lunch.

EASY SOLUTION FOR WHAT'S FOR DINNER

When I'm in a pinch, I often turn to this formula and think about how I can layer a carbohydrate with a quick-cooking protein and then top that with veggies and a boost of flavor. Often I serve these meals in a bowl, but they start with this formula.

The one-pot meal formula—aka "When In Doubt, Stir Fry".

- **Two to three parts veggie:** choose from broccoli, snap peas, bok choy, asparagus, corn, Brussels sprouts, carrots, diced eggplant, garlic, onion, bell peppers, mushrooms, parsnips, turnip, kale, green beans, peas, sprouts, celery, etc.
- **One part grain:** choose from white rice, brown rice, wild rice, rice noodles, udon noodles, vermicelli, etc.
- **One part protein:** choose from chicken, shrimp, ground turkey, ground beef, strip steak, tofu, tempeh, scrambled egg, etc.
- **Always the same:** oil, soy sauce/tamari, water/broth, vinegar, salt and pepper.
- **Optional toppings:** sliced green onions, sesame seeds, chili flakes, lime juice, avocado slices, fresh herbs.

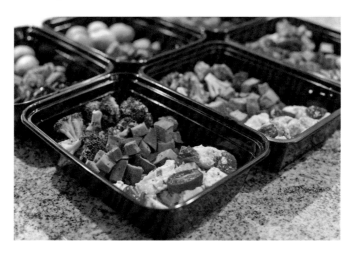

You might think about this meal formula only with Asian flavors, but I like to make it Mexican with salsa and avocado or Mediterranean using hummus as a dressing and adding walnuts and feta. Use your own favorite flavor profiles and creativity!

Breakfast for dinner is another quick dinner idea that can be pulled together easily using your stocked kitchen. An egg burrito is a quick way to get a well-balanced dinner on the table and save hundreds of calories over take-out options.

DIETITIAN-APPROVED CONVENIENCE FOODS

When you're making improvements to your diet, you might think it will take a lot of time. I recommend using certain convenience foods in your meal prep. We don't have to work harder to eat smarter. Everything we eat doesn't have to be homemade to help us reach our nutrition goals.

Here is a list of convenience foods that get the green light from most dietitians and can be used to stock your kitchen for healthy eating success.

- Stir-in spice pastes
- Fresh herb tubes
- Microwave rice and grains
- Frozen fruits and vegetables
- Whole grain breads and crackers
- Nut butter, single servings for travel
- Bone broth
- Salad dressing made with avocado oil and low sugar
- Bagged salad kits
- Pre-cut fruits and vegetables IF it makes you more likely to eat them
- Canned tuna and salmon
- Canned diced tomatoes or tomato sauce
- Frozen meals with at least 10 grams of protein, 8 grams of fiber, and low sodium
- Frozen veggie burgers
- Canned beans, low sodium preferred
- Prepared pesto sauce
- Frozen seafood
- Frozen egg bites
- String cheese
- Higher protein cereal
- Frozen edamame.

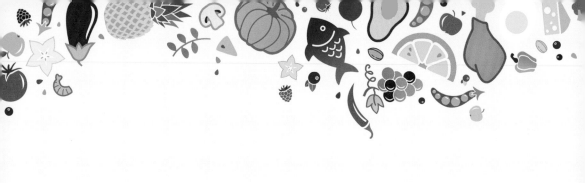

CHAPTER 8

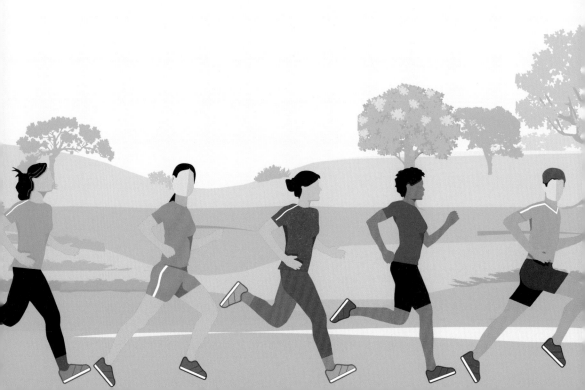

MEAL PLANS FOR POPULAR DIETS

Carissa Galloway, RDN

Just because a diet is popular doesn't mean it's right for you. Here are some popular diets that get a nod of approval from Jeff and me.

The best diet is . . . the one you stick with! Restrictive diets won't work for most people long term. It's important to develop a diet that can help you maintain healthy nutrition habits for the long term and a diet that lets you include foods that you love.

When it comes to building that diet, there is not a one-size-fits-all approach for everyone. I find that it's helpful to not only have a knowledge of basic nutrition (which you're getting in this book), but to look at other popular diets. When you look at other well-balanced diets, then you can borrow pieces that might work well for you and your family. This can be a helpful way to create your ideal diet and a healthy eating pattern that can provide you nutrients and energy for life.

Following are several popular diets that I recommend. They are all well-balanced, meaning they don't exclude any major food groups. They also are relatively easy to follow, which makes you more likely to stick with them for longer. Finally, they provide enough calories for an active lifestyle, but can be trimmed to provide a slight calorie deficit that would support steady weight loss.

MEDITERRANEAN DIET

The Mediterranean diet is constantly ranked as one of the top diets and has been ranked #1 on U.S. News's list of recommended diets. Overall, the Mediterranean diet is nutritionally sound offering diverse foods and flavors. It's also generally easy to follow and not overly restrictive. You can say that both Jeff and I have built our diets off principles of the Mediterranean diet.

The Mediterranean diet focuses on:

- Maintaining an active lifestyle
- Weight control

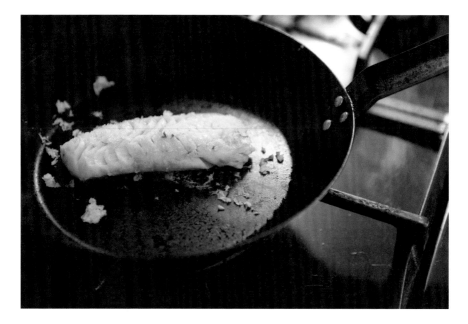

- Limiting red meat, sugar, saturated fat
- Health benefits associated with the diet may include weight loss, heart and brain health, cancer prevention, and diabetes prevention and control.

The Mediterranean diet includes:

- Olive oil, beans, nuts, legumes, seeds, herbs, and spices; you will base most meals on these
- Fruits, vegetables, and mainly whole grains
- Fish and seafood at least two times a week
- Poultry, eggs, cheese, and yogurt will be used moderately, at most at one meal daily
- Meat and sweets are used less often
- Wine is allowed in moderation
- Daily physical activity is encouraged.

Sample Mediterranean diet day:

- Breakfast—full-fat Greek yogurt with nuts, honey, and fruit
- Lunch—chickpea pita with a side salad
- Dinner—roasted white fish and olives with roasted vegetables topped with a squeeze of lemon.

THE DASH DIET

The DASH diet (which stands for Dietary Approach to Stop Hypertension) was originally created as a diet to stop high blood pressure (hypertension). While it does limit salt, it does so much more and can be a well-balanced and lower-sodium diet for anyone. Most Americans currently consume too much sodium from processed and packaged foods, and any attempt to decrease salt consumption will be beneficial for your overall health.

Along with recommending decreased sodium, the DASH diet encourages increased consumption of fruits, veggies, whole grains, lean protein, and low-fat dairy, which are high in blood pressure-deflating nutrients, such as potassium, calcium, protein, and fiber. DASH also discourages foods that are high in saturated fat, such as fatty meats, full-fat dairy foods, and tropical oils, as well as sugar-sweetened beverages and sweets. The DASH diet limits sodium at 2,300 milligrams a day for some, and about 1,500 milligrams for others at higher risk for hypertension. The DASH diet will require some label reading. This will help you seek out lower-sodium foods and see what foods you're currently eating that are too high in sodium.

The DASH diet recommends small dietary changes that can be sustainable rather than dramatic changes. I wholeheartedly agree with this approach.

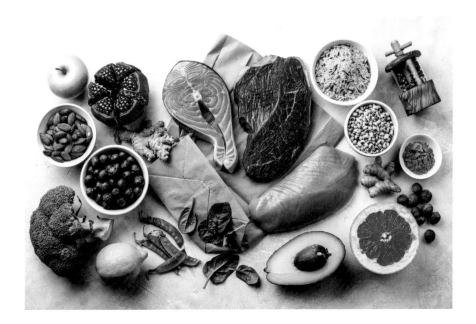

Small changes recommended with the DASH diet include:

- Adding one vegetable or fruit serving to every meal
- Introducing two or more meat-free meals each week
- Using herbs and spices to make food tastier without the salt
- Snack swaps like almonds or pecans instead of a bag of chips
- Switching from white flour to whole-wheat flour when possible
- Taking a 15-minute walk after lunch or dinner (or both).

Foods encouraged on the DASH diet include:

- Fruits
- Vegetables
- Whole grains
- Low-fat dairy
- Lean meats like chicken breast, turkey breast, lean cuts of pork or red meat
- Seafood
- Nuts, seeds, legumes
- Plant-based oils, such as olive oil or avocado oil.

Foods to avoid on the DASH diet include:

- Sugar, candy, cookies, cakes
- Full-fat dairy and cheese
- Enriched grains
- Processed or convenience foods with high sodium levels
- Alcohol.

Sample DASH diet day:

- Breakfast—Old Fashioned Oats made with low-fat milk, fresh berries, and honey
- Lunch—hummus and veggie sandwich on whole grain toast
- Snack(s)—small orange and sunflower seeds, grapes with Romano cheese
- Dinner—shrimp and broccoli with whole grain pasta in olive oil and garlic.

THE FLEXITARIAN DIET

A diet that has increased in popularity in the last decade is the "Flexitarian diet." What I love is what the name implies. It's flexible! It allows you to make a shift to more plant-based meals while not feeling guilty for enjoying lean meats or seafood in moderation too. The diet is mostly vegetarian but allows for flexibility. It's recommended that you start with two meat-free days and increase that number to as many meat-free days as possible.

The Flexitarian diet focuses on "adding in" foods as opposed to just focusing on taking meat out of your diet.

Five groups of foods to include in your diet:

- The "new meat" (non-meat proteins like beans, peas, or eggs)
- Fruits and veggies
- Whole grains
- Dairy
- Spice and flavor from things like citrus juice or herbs.

Sample Flexitarian diet day:

- Breakfast—avocado toast with sprouted whole grain toast, avocado, spinach, and egg
- Lunch—bowl with canned tuna or chickpeas, chopped kale or tomatoes, roasted sweet potato cubes, and ranch dressing
- Dinner—tacos with seasoned white fish or lentils, corn tortillas, cabbage slaw, guacamole, and salsa
- Snack—apple and pecans and/or cucumber sticks and hummus.

Sometimes we learn best from others. I have found with clients and myself it can be insightful to see what others eat and use that to get ideas for balancing your own nutrition. Here is a "typical" day of eating from your two authors!

JEFF'S NUTRITION ON AN AVERAGE DAY

6 a.m. Out of bed, pour cold press coffee that has brewed overnight

7 a.m. Finish 12 ounces of coffee, poured cup #2 while answering emails that came in overnight

8 a.m. Eat an orange, banana, or another fruit, or bowl of Great Grains cereal, with blueberries or grapes

8:30 to 9:30 a.m. Morning workout

9:30 to 10 a.m. Eat a 200-calorie snack or an energy bar, Great Grains cereal, or another carbohydrate snack, and drink 12 ounces of water

10 to 11:30 a.m. Drink 12 ounces of seltzer water while working (on cross-training days, do 30 minutes of elliptical or rower)

11:30 to 12 noon Lunch with 12 ounces of seltzer water and one of the following:

- Baked potato with lentils or black beans
- Salmon or chicken breast sandwich
- Cooked vegetables with rice or baked potato
- Baked beans or black beans with coleslaw or collard greens.

2 to 2:30 p.m. Twelve ounces of seltzer water, snack on one of the following:

- Banana with peanut butter
- Tortilla with peanut butter and pickles
- Small bowl of almonds or peanuts
- Bowl of Great Grains cereal.

4 p.m. Twelve-ounce glass of water or 12 ounces of coffee, snack on one of the following:

- Black beans or baked beans with coleslaw
- Baked potato with coleslaw.

5 p.m. Second workout

6 p.m. Snack of watermelon, banana, grapes, 8 to 12 ounces of cold water

7 p.m. Dinner with 12 ounces of seltzer water and one of the following:

- Mixed salad with salmon or other fish and baked potato or rice
- Cooked vegetables with grilled chicken with baked potato or pasta
- Bean dish: soup, chili, casserole with mixed salad, rice, or whole grain bread
- Vegetables: collard greens, black eyed peas, broccoli, cauliflower, etc., with rice or whole grain bread or potato
- Pasta with either grilled chicken, grilled fish, or vegetables
- Dessert—banana, grapes, watermelon, peaches, etc.
- Medicinal dose after dinner—a glass of red wine or a glass of IPA, every other night.

CARISSA'S NUTRITION ON AN AVERAGE DAY

8 a.m. Coffee with cream and one scoop of collagen

9 to 9:30 a.m. Frozen protein waffle topped with peanut butter, Lite syrup, and fresh berries

Morning snack—Mamma Chia pouch or handful of dry cheerios

12 to 1 p.m. Lunch—usually leftovers from the night before or an Amy's frozen meal

Afternoon snack—Apple and later a small cheese and cracker plate or handful of pistachios

Dinner—Baked salmon, ½ cup rice and quinoa blend, sautéed spinach, 1 ounce feta cheese.

You may have noticed that many of those diets suggest similar principles. Many of those principles were also discussed earlier in this book. Nutrition can seem complicated, but a few basic ideas can evolve into a lifelong healthy diet for you and your family. I hope this chapter has given you a few ideas of what your nutrition philosophy might be and how to use this knowledge to shape a healthy you and a healthier diet.

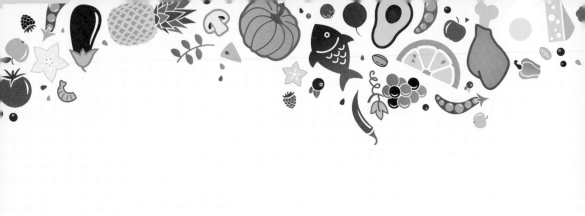

CHAPTER 9

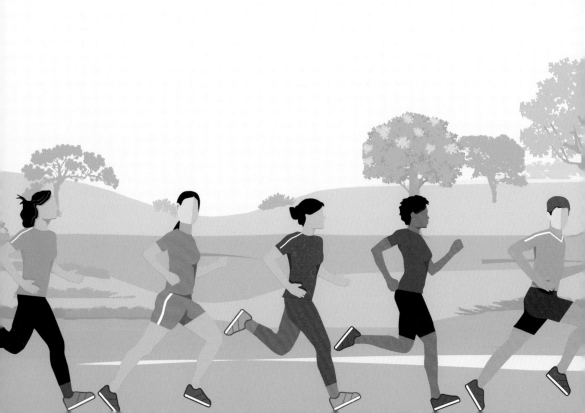

CARISSA'S RECIPES

MAKE-AHEAD BREAKFASTS

PUMPKIN-BAKED OATMEAL

This is a great make-ahead option to provide a heart-healthy fiber-packed breakfast that's ready quickly in the morning. It will not be overly sweet, so we add a little maple syrup and top with peanut butter.

 BONUS RECIPE: OVERNIGHT OATS

INGREDIENTS

- 3 cups Old Fashioned Oats
- 2 teaspoons baking powder
- ½ teaspoon salt
- 1 tablespoon + cinnamon (add more to your taste)
- 2 teaspoons pumpkin pie spice
- 2 cups plain almond milk (can use other type of milk)
- 3 tablespoons egg white substitute
- 1 6 oz container Greek yogurt
- 1 cup canned pure pumpkin (not pumpkin pie filling)
- ⅓ cup slivered almonds
- ¾ cup coconut flakes

DIRECTIONS

1. Preheat oven to 400°F.
2. In a bowl, mix dry ingredients—oats, baking powder, salt, cinnamon, pumpkin pie spice.
3. In another bowl, mix wet ingredients—milk, egg white, yogurt, pumpkin. Combine the wet and dry ingredients.
4. Add almonds and coconut.
5. Pour into a greased 9 × 13″ casserole dish and bake uncovered for 20 minutes.
6. Remove from oven and stir. Bake uncovered an additional 20 minutes.

HASH BROWN AND EGG BIRDS' NESTS

Most Americans don't get enough protein at breakfast, so these are a great make-ahead way to balance protein and necessary carbohydrates in the morning, as well as a potassium boost from the potatoes. This makes 6 muffins, 3 muffins per serving.

INGREDIENTS
- olive oil spray
- 4 cups of shredded potatoes
- 1 teaspoon garlic powder
- salt and pepper to taste
- 5 liquid egg whites
- ½ chopped onion
- ½ cup diced bell peppers
- ¼ cup shredded cheddar cheese
- 4 teaspoons salsa

DIRECTIONS
1. Preheat oven to 375°F.
2. Spray a muffin tin with oil or non-stick spray.
3. Shred potatoes using cheese grater or use pre-packaged shredded potatoes. Combine potatoes with garlic powder, salt, and pepper.
4. Evenly distribute potato mixture in muffin tins and press the mixture in the middle using a spoon so that it forms a nest.
5. Bake for 30 to 35 minutes or until golden brown with crisp edges.
6. When nests are baking, combine eggs, onions, peppers, cheese, and salsa in a bowl.
7. When nests are golden brown, remove from oven and fill with ¼ cup of egg mixture.
8. Bake for 15 to 20 minutes until the eggs are cooked.

MEDITERRANEAN BREAKFAST HASH

Serving Size: 2

INGREDIENTS

- 2 teaspoons extra virgin olive oil
- 2 russet potatoes, diced
- ½ cup red onion, chopped
- 3 garlic cloves, chopped
- ½ cup canned chickpeas, drained and rinsed
- 3 cups baby spinach (can use frozen but make sure to squeeze the water out and only use ½ cup)
- 1 tsp dried oregano
- 1 tsp paprika
- salt and pepper
- ¼ cup chopped grape tomatoes
- 4 eggs, whisked in a bowl
- ½ cup crumbled feta
- ½ cup chopped fresh parsley, stems removed
- 1 lemon

DIRECTIONS

1. Heat 1 teaspoon olive oil in a large cast-iron skillet on medium-high heat. Add the potatoes and onions and cook for 3 to 5 minutes. Add the garlic and cook for another 3 to 5 minutes, stirring frequently until the potatoes are tender. If the potatoes brown or form a golden crust, that is ok and quite delicious!
2. Reduce heat to medium. Add ½ teaspoon of extra virgin olive oil. Add the drained chickpeas, spinach, dried oregano, paprika, salt and pepper. Stir to combine. Cook for 5 minutes or until the spinach is wilted. Add chopped tomatoes and cook for 2 more minutes. Push hash mixture to the outside of the pan leaving space for the eggs.
3. Add ½ teaspoon of olive oil to the pan and add the eggs to the middle of the pan. Cook eggs on medium-low heat, gently pulling across the eggs with a spatula as they begin to set. Continue pulling, lifting, and folding the eggs until no liquid remains and they are cooked to your preference. Once the eggs are cooked, fold them into the hash mixture.
4. Remove the potato hash from the heat and add the feta and parsley. Slice the lemon in half and squeeze on top of the dish. Enjoy!

SUPER SMOOTHIES

PURPLE POTATO POWER SMOOTHIE

Are potatoes in a smoothie interesting? Yes! But they give you potassium and quick digesting carbohydrates, which are perfect with your morning energy boost.

INGREDIENTS
- 4 small 2" purple potatoes
- 1 small banana (can be frozen)
- 1 cup pomegranate juice
- 2 tablespoons plain or vanilla whey protein powder
- 1 teaspoon honey
- 1 handful ice cubes

DIRECTIONS
1. Bring a pot of water to boil. Once boiling, add small purple potatoes and cook until soft, about 15 minutes. You can also microwave potatoes. Pierce with a fork and microwave until soft for 4 to 6 minutes.
2. Blend all ingredients including potatoes in a blender until smooth.
3. Taste and adjust seasoning as desired. Add more honey or banana to sweeten. Add more ice to thicken.

TURMERIC RECOVERY SMOOTHIE

This is a great post-workout smoothie to jumpstart your recovery. You're not only getting protein but powerful anti-inflammatory compounds from curcumin. Curcumin is the main active ingredient in turmeric and a very strong antioxidant. Curcumin fights inflammation in various ways at molecular level, resulting in reduced inflammation throughout the body. Don't skip the pepper! Just a dash of pepper will boost your body's absorption of the turmeric by 1,000.

INGREDIENTS
- 1 banana
- 1 cup frozen mango
- ¾ cup plain kefir
- ½ to 1 teaspoon turmeric
- dash pepper

DIRECTIONS
1. Place all ingredients into a blender and mix until smooth.
2. Add ice if desired.

CHOCOLATE GREEN SMOOTHIE

We all need more greens in our diet and adding a bit into a smoothie is a great way to get more. I never make a smoothie without spinach, however, it can turn it an odd color, so this is a great starter spinach smoothie recipe for the skeptics.

INGREDIENTS
- 1 cup almond milk (or milk of your choice)
- 1 cup baby spinach
- ¼ teaspoon cinnamon
- 1 scoop chocolate protein powder
- 1 frozen banana
- 1 teaspoon nut butter

DIRECTIONS
1. Place all ingredients into a blender and mix until smooth.
2. Add ice if desired.
3. Garnish with extra cinnamon if desired.

FISH IS YOUR FRIEND

BAKED PESTO SALMON

Getting in two servings of omega-3-rich salmon a week doesn't need to be hard. Our family loves the ease of this sheet pan meal and the rich flavor the pesto adds to the salmon.

 BAKED PESTO SALMON DEMO

INGREDIENTS

- non-stick cooking spray
- 4 6-oz salmon fillets, if skin on, place skin side down
- 6 tablespoons pesto
- ⅓ cup fresh breadcrumbs
- ⅓ cup freshly grated parmesan cheese
- 1½ cup broccoli florets
- 1 tablespoon extra virgin olive oil

DIRECTIONS

1. Preheat the oven to 350°F.
2. Place a piece of tin foil on a rimmed baking sheet. Spray with non-stick cooking spray. Place salmon fillets on the baking sheet leaving space for the broccoli.
3. Spoon 1½ tablespoons of pesto over each fillet and spread it evenly.
4. In a small bowl, combine the breadcrumbs and parmesan cheese until evenly distributed. Top each of the salmon fillets with equal amounts breadcrumb mixture.
5. In a small bowl, combine the broccoli and olive oil. Place on the sheet pan around the salmon.
6. Cook the salmon for 15 to 20 minutes for medium. To get the crust a golden brown, turn the oven to broil and heat for 45 seconds to 1½ minutes with the salmon about 5" away from the heating element. When broiling, watch closely so it does not burn.

ALMOND-CRUSTED TILAPIA

The seafood dish requires less than 10 minutes of prep and can be served as a low-carb dinner, on top of a fresh salad, or with a simple side like a 90-second rice packet. You can also swap other proteins with this method like chicken, salmon, or mahi-mahi.

INGREDIENTS
- non-stick cooking spray
- 1 cup slivered almonds, divided in 2 parts
- ¼ cup ground flaxseed (you can substitute flour, but I recommend the flax for nutrition benefits)
- 2 tablespoon olive oil or oil of your choice
- ½ teaspoon salt
- 1 teaspoon garlic powder
- 4 6-oz tilapia fillets
- ¼ cup grated parmesan cheese
- sliced lemon for garnish and final seasoning (optional)
- Ground flaxseeds

DIRECTIONS
1. Preheat oven to BROIL.
2. Spray a large, rimmed baking sheet with cooking spray. Set aside.
3. Combine half of the slivered almonds (½ cup) with the ground flaxseed or flour in a shallow bowl. Set aside.
4. Combine olive oil, salt, and garlic powder in a small bowl. Brush the mixture on both sides of the fish.
5. Place the fish on the prepared baking sheet, bottom side UP, and broil for 4 minutes.
6. Flip the fish over, sprinkle with ground flaxseeds, parmesan cheese, and almonds, and return to the broiler for about 3 to 5 more minutes. Fish is done when the topping is golden brown and the fish flakes easily with a fork.
7. Garnish with lemon wedges.

SESAME-GINGER TUNA SALAD

This salad is an easy way to get those essential omega-3s in your diet, and because you're using canned tuna, there's no prep time.

INGREDIENTS

- 2 5 to 6-oz cans chunk light tuna, drained
- 1 cup sugar snap peas, sliced
- 2 tablespoons chopped green onion
- 3 tablespoons canola oil
- 2 tablespoons reduced sodium soy sauce
- 1 tablespoon toasted sesame oil
- 1¼ tsp sugar
- 1 tsp grated fresh ginger
- 6 cups shredded romaine lettuce or napa cabbage
- ¼ cup chopped cilantro
- 2 tablespoons toasted sesame seeds
- ¼ cup rice wine vinegar

DIRECTIONS

1. Combine tuna, peas, and green onion in a bowl.
2. Whisk canola oil, soy sauce, sesame oil, sugar, rice wine vinegar and ginger in a bowl. Add 3 tablespoons of mixture to the tuna bowl, toss to combine.
3. Put 1½ cups of shredded lettuce on a plate, top with ½ cup of the dressed tuna mixture, and drizzle with about 2 tablespoons of remaining dressing. Top with toasted sesame seeds.

DINNERS THAT MAKE GREAT LEFTOVERS

CHICKEN ENCHILADA CASSEROLE

INGREDIENTS
- non-stick cooking spray
- 1 package chicken breasts, cooked and shredded
- 1 tablespoon extra virgin olive oil
- 1 medium onion, diced
- 1 medium zucchini, diced
- 2 19-oz cans black beans, rinsed
- 1 14-oz can diced tomatoes, drained
- 1½ cups corn, frozen (thawed) or fresh
- 1 teaspoon ground cumin
- 1 package Sazón GOYA seasoning (optional)
- ½ teaspoon salt
- 12 corn tortillas, quartered
- 1 19-oz can mild red or green enchilada sauce
- 1¼ cups shredded reduced-fat Cheddar cheese (optional)

DIRECTIONS
1. Preheat oven to 400°F. Lightly coat a 9 × 13" baking pan with cooking spray.
2. Use poached or Slow cooker cooked chicken breasts. Shred chicken.
3. Heat oil in a large non-stick skillet over a medium-high heat. Add onion and cook, stirring often, until starting to brown for about 5 minutes. Stir in zucchini, beans, tomatoes, corn, cumin, GOYA, and salt, and cook, stirring occasionally, until the vegetables are heated through, about 3 minutes.
4. Scatter half the tortilla pieces in the pan. Top with half the vegetable mixture, half the enchilada sauce, and half the cheese. Repeat with one more layer of tortillas, vegetables, sauce, and cheese. Cover with foil.
5. Bake the casserole for 15 minutes. Remove the foil and continue baking until the casserole is bubbling around the edges and the cheese is melted for about 10 minutes more.

SKINNY TURKEY LASAGNA

This is a family favorite recipe that's recently been our Christmas night dinner. It's comfort food, you can make it ahead, it makes great leftovers. What's there not to love?

INGREDIENTS

- 1 zucchini diced
- 1lb lean ground turkey
- 1 15-oz can crushed tomatoes
- 1 small can tomato sauce
- ½ cup water
- 3 teaspoons oregano
- 1 teaspoon red pepper flakes
- 2 teaspoons Italian seasoning
- fresh ground pepper
- 1 teaspoon garlic powder
- 1 teaspoon onion powder
- 1 teaspoon salt
- 1 white onion diced
- 2 teaspoons garlic
- extra virgin olive oil
- 2 eggs
- 15 oz part-skim ricotta cheese
- ¼ cup shredded Italian cheese (additional cheese to top lasagna if desired)
- ½ cup fresh chopped parsley (keep some for garnish)
- 9 whole wheat lasagna noodles—uncooked

DIRECTIONS

1. Dice zucchini and cook in a skillet coated with non-stick cooking spray. While the zucchini softens, add the crushed tomato, tomato sauce, water, and all the spices to a different large pot. Adjust seasonings to taste. Bring to a simmer.
2. Add softened zucchini to tomato sauce.
3. Sauté onions and garlic in a little olive oil until tender. Add the turkey to the pan and cook until no longer pink, breaking it up into the smallest pieces you can.
4. Add the turkey and onion mixture to the tomato sauce. Simmer on low for 1 to 2 hours. Adjust spices as needed.
5. In a bowl beat 2 eggs. Add the ricotta, shredded cheese, parsley, salt, and pepper. Mix well.
6. Using a 9 × 13" pan begin the lasagna-forming process.
7. Cover the bottom of the pan with 1 cup of sauce. Layer 3 noodles. Top with sauce then add half the ricotta mixture. Add 3 noodles. Top with sauce, then add the remaining ricotta mixture evenly. Top with 3 noodles and top with remaining sauce. Add additional shredded cheese on the top. I don't add a lot of cheese because I find it doesn't add that much flavor compared with the extra calories.
8. Cover with foil and bake in a 350°F oven for 50 minutes.
9. Remove foil and bake an additional 10 minutes or broil to achieve desired "brownness" on cheese. I like browned cheese . . . when I eat cheese.
10. Let it cool.
11. Top with fresh parsley and enjoy.

TERIYAKI PINEAPPLE MEATBALLS

These are a creative twist on a meal prep favorite and are great as an appetizer for entertaining or game watching! If you want to make these as an appetizer, I would recommend making the meatballs smaller. You would need to reduce the cooking time to 15 to 20 minutes until cooked through. I like to serve them with fresh pineapple on a skewer for a fun, flavorful bite.

INGREDIENTS
- Non-stick cooking spray
- 1 lb ground turkey
- ¾ cup panko
- 1 egg, beaten
- 2 teaspoons minced fresh ginger
- 2 cloves minced garlic
- 2 tablespoons minced green onions (scallions)
- ½ cup can crushed pineapple, juices drained
- 2 teaspoons teriyaki sauce (any brand, you can use low sodium)
- ½ teaspoon salt
- ¼ teaspoon black pepper
- Rice or lettuce wrap (to serve, optional)

DIRECTIONS
1. Preheat oven to 400°F. Spray a foil-lined baking sheet with cooking spray.
2. In a large bowl, combine ground turkey, panko, milk, egg, ginger, garlic, green onions, pineapple, salt, pepper, and teriyaki sauce.
3. Stir until combined.
4. Roll the mixture into 1¼ to 1½" meatballs.
5. Place meatballs onto baking sheet and bake for 25 minutes or until slightly brown on top.
6. Garnish with green onions.
7. Serve on rice, lettuce wrap, or as an appetizer.

SLOW COOKER CREATIONS

SALSA SLOW COOKER CHICKEN

 SALSA SLOW COOKER CHICKEN DEMO

This recipe is a go-to at our house for when we have guests coming. It's easy and it will be ready when your guests arrive. I make it as part of a taco or taco bowl "bar" and allow my guests to customize their bowls. This salsa chicken also works great for meal prep. It can be used for several days in a variety of Mexican-inspired dishes like burritos, quesadillas, and even nachos!

INGREDIENTS

- 1.5 lb. boneless, skinless chicken breasts, trimmed of any fat
- 1 cup salsa

DIRECTIONS

1. Add chicken to the slow cooker. Top with salsa.
2. Cover the slow cooker and cook on high 3 to 4 hours or low 6 to 8 hours. Once the chicken is cooked shred with a fork and mix with salsa.

SLOW COOKER CHICKEN TIKKA MASALA

This dish allows you to harness the anti-inflammatory power of turmeric. Chicken with sauce works great in the Slow cooker because it prevents the chicken from drying out, and I love the bold flavors and a tikka masala.

INGREDIENTS

- 1 15-oz can full-fat coconut milk
- 1 15-oz can tomato sauce
- 2 tablespoons garam masala
- 1 teaspoon ground cumin
- ½ teaspoon ground turmeric
- ½ teaspoon garlic powder
- ¼ teaspoon ground ginger
- ¼ teaspoon salt
- 2 large red potatoes, chopped into 1" chunks
- 1 onion, diced
- 1.5 lb. boneless, skinless chicken breast
- Rice, quinoa, and naan bread to serve.

DIRECTIONS

1. Place coconut milk, tomato sauce, spices, and seasonings into your slow cooker and stir.
2. Then, add in the chopped potatoes and onion.
3. Add the chicken to the slow cooker and cover with the sauce.
4. Cover the slow cooker and cook on high for 3 to 4 hours or on low for 6 to 8 hours.
5. Once the chicken is fully cooked, you can shred and combine with the sauce. If you prefer chicken chunks, then remove the chicken from the sauce and cut into desired size pieces. Return to the slow cooker and combine with the sauce.
6. Serve over rice or quinoa or with naan.

SLOW COOKER APPLE CINNAMON OATMEAL

As a dietitian, I know the health benefits of oatmeal. As a busy mom, I know oatmeal can take longer to prep in the morning. Barb Galloway starts most days with oatmeal, which shows that this is a great way to combine a healthy superfood with meal prep. Make this on Sunday afternoons and portion out for quick weekday breakfasts.

INGREDIENTS

- 1.5 cups steel-cut oats
- 3 cups milk of your choice
- 3 cups water
- ½ cup real maple syrup
- 2 teaspoons cinnamon
- 2 large apples, diced
- ¼ teaspoon salt
- To serve: nut butter, fruit, nut pieces, spoonful of vanilla yogurt (optional)

DIRECTIONS

1. Place oats, milk, water, maple syrup, cinnamon, apples, and salt in a slow cooker and mix.
2. Cover and cook on low for around 6 to 8 hours or on high for 3 to 4 hours. Aim to stir hourly throughout the cooking process.
3. Serve with nut butter, more fruit, nut pieces, or a spoonful of vanilla yogurt.
4. If you need to reheat it, add a splash of water and microwave for 60 to 90 seconds.

VERY EASY VEGETARIAN

BLACK BEAN RICE BOWL

This is a favorite weeknight meal in our house. It can come together with just pantry staples, and it's filling and flavorful! We use a variety of microwaveable lime rice, but you can use whatever rice you prefer. We also serve it with a few tortilla chips to add texture. Makes 2 servings.

BLACK BEAN RICE BOWL DEMO

INGREDIENTS
- 1 package microwaveable lime rice
- 1 can of black beans, drained and rinsed
- ¼ cup salsa
- ½ cup sliced grape tomatoes
- ½ cup diced red or yellow bell peppers
- ½ avocado sliced
- ½ cup shredded cheddar cheese
- optional: cilantro, diced white onions, jalapeño, tortilla chips

DIRECTIONS
1. Cook rice according to package directions.
2. Add drained and rinsed beans to a microwave-safe container and heat to your desired temperature, for about 75 seconds.
3. Build your bowl the way you want! I recommend starting with the rice at the bottom of the bowl and layer with beans then the toppings.

BUILD-YOUR-OWN GREEK BOWL

If this recipe seems like the one above it, that's because it is! The bowl method is a formula that works well for vegetarian dishes and is perfect for busy weeknights or a work-day lunch. The key is to layer a carbohydrate, a vegetarian protein source, vegetables, a creamy component, and something for texture. This recipe is our family's traditional Greek bowl, but you can make any tweaks or additions to fit your palate and what's in your kitchen. This can be served hot or cold. Makes 2 servings.

INGREDIENTS
- 1 cup cooked quinoa (can substitute rice, orzo pasta, farro, sorghum)
- 1 16 oz can of beans of your choice, drained and rinsed (for the Greek bowl I prefer Great Northern or garbanzo beans)
- ½ cup of hummus
- ½ cup sliced grape tomatoes
- ½ cup diced cucumbers
- ¼ cup olives
- ½ cup crumbled feta cheese
- ½ cup toasted walnuts

DIRECTIONS
1. Prepare your grain of choice.
2. Add drained and rinsed beans to a microwave-safe container and heat to your desired temperature, about 75 seconds.
3. Build your bowl the way you want! I recommend starting with the quinoa at the bottom of the bowl, and layer with chickpeas, then toppings.

VEGETABLE FRITTATA

If you're new to the concept of adding in meatless meals, then a frittata is a great way to start. Eggs are a high-protein food that's familiar to meat eaters. Eggs are also affordable, and a frittata is an easy one-pan dish that adds veggies into a savory, filling dish. This is also a good way to use up leftover vegetables in your pantry. Feel free to make substitutions to the recipe to use whatever vegetables are in your house.

INGREDIENTS
- 6 whole eggs
- ¼ cup milk of your choice
- 1 cup shredded cheddar cheese
- salt and pepper
- 1 tablespoon avocado oil
- ¼ cup chopped onions
- 1 cup chopped mushrooms
- 1 cup sliced spinach
- 10 stalks chopped asparagus
- ½ cup sliced grape tomatoes

DIRECTIONS
1. Preheat oven to 425°F.
2. Whisk the eggs and milk in a large bowl.
3. Add in the cheese and stir. Season with salt and pepper.
4. Heat the oil in an oven-safe pan or cast-iron skillet. Add the vegetables and cook for 4 to 6 minutes until soft.
5. Pour the egg mixture on top of the vegetables. Add sliced tomatoes to the top.
6. Bake uncovered for 10 to 15 minutes. It is done when the center is set and does not jiggle.

FAMILY FAVORITE RECIPES

CHICKEN MANDARIN ORANGE SALAD

My Mom makes great salads. They take up an entire mixing bowl and they're packed with flavor, texture, nutrients, and always homemade dressings. Homemade dressings are not hard to make. They are far superior nutritionally to store-bought dressing especially when it comes to added sugar and the use of oils like soybean oil. Plus they are usually more affordable to make at home too.

INGREDIENTS

For the dressing:

- 6 tablespoons orange juice (fresh squeezed or store bought)
- 1 to 2 tablespoons orange zest
- 4 tablespoons seasoned rice vinegar (plain or roasted garlic)
- ¼ to ½ teaspoon garlic powder (to taste)
- salt (to taste)
- 3 tablespoons extra virgin olive oil

For the Salad:

- 8 oz or to your liking, spinach (or your favorite greens or mix)
- 1½ cup diced leftover or pan seared (cooked) chicken
- 1 can, 45 oz no-sugar-added mandarin orange segments, drained
- ¼ cup chopped cilantro
- 1 avocado: pitted, peeled and diced
- sliced almonds for garnish
- fresh cracked pepper (optional)

DIRECTIONS

For the salad dressing:

1. Mix first 5 ingredients together in a jar. Shake to mix.
2. Taste and adjust as needed.
3. Add extra virgin olive oil and shake to mix.
4. Cool in refrigerator until you are ready to serve the salad.

For the salad:

1. Plate the ingredients for serving starting with the greens, then the chicken and mandarin oranges, next the cilantro, place the avocado.
2. Top it all off with the sliced almond garnish and cracked black pepper to taste.

SMOKY PAPRIKA VINAIGRETTE

This is a creative dressing that can add big flavor to a salad, and it's a great way to use up leftover grilled meats or vegetables. The paprika boosts anti-inflammatory properties. My mom created this recipe after I had my first child, Claire. She would make me dinner each week, and this salad dressing was requested a lot to support healing and get a nutritious meal in me, which, as new moms might remember, isn't easy to do those first few weeks. This recipe makes enough dressing for two servings, so double the recipe if you are serving more. I like to serve this salad with grilled chicken or shrimp over dark, leafy greens, shredded carrots, avocado, feta cheese, and crunchy wonton bits.

INGREDIENTS
- juice of 1 fresh lemon (no seeds) or 1 tablespoon lemon concentrate
- zest of 1 lemon (optional)
- 4 tablespoons of your favorite vinegar (rice, wine, apple cider, etc.)
- 1 tablespoon sugar
- 1 teaspoon garlic powder
- 1 teaspoon smoky paprika
- 2 teaspoons onion powder
- ¼ teaspoon fresh cracked pepper
- ¼ teaspoon cinnamon
- ¼ teaspoon ground ginger
- 2 tablespoons extra virgin olive oil

DIRECTIONS
1. Mix all ingredients together except for the olive oil in a jar with a lid. I use recycled sauce jars with similar lids to a canning jar . . . recycle . . . re-use!
2. Allow the spices to bloom in the acids for a few minutes before adding the olive oil.
3. Add the oil to the jar, add the lid, and shake. Note: this will be thicker with spice than any store-bought vinaigrette.

TURKEY BURGERS WITH CHIA SEEDS

For the many of Americans that don't eat enough seafood, chia seeds are something I frequently to add into their diets. Chia seeds are rich in omega 3s, antioxidants, and fiber. Usually chia seeds are added into breakfast items, such as oatmeal or muffins, so this recipe, inspired by Barb Galloway, is a great way to work them into dinner too. Plus it adds moisture to lean ground turkey, which can otherwise easily dry out if overcooked. These turkey burgers freeze well. Make extra and freeze the uncooked patties for a quick weeknight meal.

INGREDIENTS

- 1½ tablespoons chia seeds
- ½ cup water
- ½ medium yellow onion chopped
- 1 tablespoon minced garlic
- 1 tablespoon extra virgin olive oil (only if caramelizing onions)
- 1 lb lean ground turkey breast
- ½ cup grated carrot
- 1 tablespoon finely chopped parsley
- 1 teaspoon Trader Joe's Everyday Seasoning
- ½ teaspoon Worcestershire sauce
- ½ teaspoon salt

DIRECTIONS

1. Combine chia seeds and ½ cup water. Stir constantly, for ½ to 1 minute. Then let the seeds set for at least 15 minutes before using in the recipe.
2. Optional step: caramelize onions in a small sauté pan if desired. Add garlic when the onions are at your desired level on doneness and cook for 1 to 2 more minutes until the garlic is fragrant. Allow the mixture to cool before adding it to the ground turkey in the next step.
3. In a medium-sized mixing bowl, add ground turkey, onion, garlic, grated carrot, chia seeds, and other seasonings. Combine well.
4. Form into 3½ to 4" patties that are about ½" thick. Cook in a sauté pan or on the grill for 4 to 5 minutes per side or until the insides measure 165°F.

A NOTE FROM CARISSA

As we close out this book, I wanted to acknowledge Jeff. He has motivated hundreds of thousands of people to get moving with his run-walk-run method. He's changed lives, and if you've picked up this book, it's likely he's changed yours.

The run-walk-run method is based on research and Jeff educates those who use his method about why it works. Once they "get" why it works, they're more likely to stick with it and thus see the amazing results.

That's why this book is so rooted in education. My goal is to give you the "why" to make better food choices. In simply picking foods that have more benefits to your body, you will be able to see changes in your nutrition, weight, energy, and performance. You will have made those choices not because you were forced to but because you knew that the outcome of those choices was beneficial to you. The end goal of this nutrition education and this book is that you will NEVER DIET AGAIN. You'll make smarter food choices, feel good about those choices, and as such, be motivated to make them again and again.

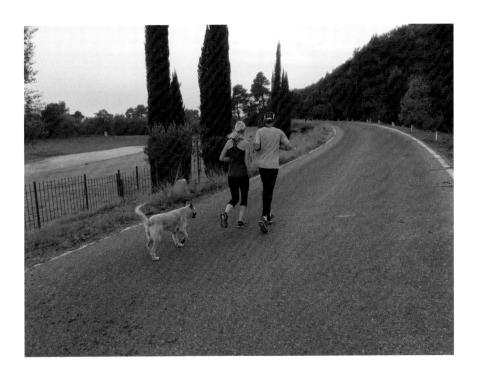

CREDITS

Cover & interior design: Anja Elsen
Layout: DiTech Publishing Services, www.ditechpubs.com
Cover photo: © AdobeStock
Interior photos: Introduction and A Note From Carissa images courtesy of Carissa
Galloway and Jeff Galloway; all other images © AdobeStock
QR videos: Courtesy of Carissa Galloway
Managing editor: Elizabeth Evans
Copy editor: Sarah Tomblin, www.sarahtomblinediting.com

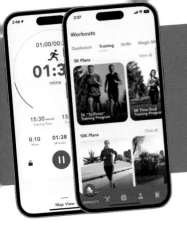

OUR BEST
FEATURES

Magic Mile Test

No need to guess how fast to run when Jeff's Magic Mile helps you dial in the perfect pace for you.

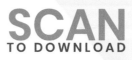

Custom Plans

Programs for any event and fitness level.

Meal Plan

Healthy meals to power your training.

Expert Advice

Daily guidance every step of the way to the finish line.

Complete Control

Customize your workout on the fly to match your needs.

Drills for Skills

Improve your running strength, form and speed.

Track

Track your workouts to see your progress.